Bircher-Benner Nutrition Plan For Prostate Problems

Other Bircher-Benner Health Guides:

Bircher-Benner Arthritis and Rheumatism Nutrition Plan
Bircher-Benner Keep-Slim Nutrition Plan
Bircher-Benner Nutrition Plan for Diabetics
Bircher-Benner Nutrition Plan for Digestive Problems
Bircher-Benner Nutrition Plan for Headache and Migraine Patients
Bircher-Benner Nutrition Plan for High Blood Pressure Problems
Bircher-Benner Nutrition Plan for Liver and Gallbladder Problems
Bircher-Benner Nutrition Plan for Skin Problems
Bircher-Benner Raw Food and Juices Nutrition Plan
Bircher-Benner Salt-Free Nutrition Plan

Bircher-Benner Nutrition Plan For Prostate Problems

A Comprehensive Guide With Suggestions for Diet Menus and Recipes

Translated by Kenneth C. Taylor

By the staff of the Bircher-Benner Clinic:

Medical/Dietetic Section:
D. Liechti-v. Brasch, M.D.,
P. F. Boesch, M.D.,
S. Grieder-Dopheide, M.D.

•

Physiological/Chemical Section:
Alfred Kunz-Bircher, Ph.D.

•

Menus and Recipes:
Ruth Kunz-Bircher, M.D.
(head of the Bircher-Benner Clinic)

•

Edited by *Ralph Bircher, M.D.*

NASH PUBLISHING • LOS ANGELES

Library of Congress Catalog Card Number: 72-81862
Standard Book Number: 8402-8046-7

Published simultaneously in the United States and
Canada by Nash Publishing Corporation,
9255 Sunset Boulevard, Los Angeles, California 90069.

Printed in the United States of America.

First Printing.

In the nineteenth century, Dr. M. Bircher-Benner established a kind of clinic that had never existed before: a clinic that would take into account the whole man, both body and soul, not only the patient's disease; a clinic that would use an intelligent patient as a co-worker in a total therapeutic effort; a clinic that would use the total knowledge of modern medicine to support the "internal physician"—the autonomous healing forces and healing system of the body—and in every case make the healing effects of dietetic therapy and one's life-style the basis of a total health plan; a clinic that, in addition to eliminating immediate ailments, would bring about a new, tougher, more satisfying and creative health of body and soul for the patient.

The private clinic founded in 1897 by Dr. Bircher-Benner is still operated today for that purpose.

Preface

Prostatic hypertrophy affects a considerable number of men in about their 50th year of life and leads to a painful obstruction of micturition with occasional sudden cystoplegia. In addition, this hypertrophy may cause many unpleasant or even perilous symptoms in the prostate region such as cystitis; severe kidney damage due to the pressure from urinary congestion, which can imperil the circulation due to high blood pressure; and even uremia with threatening phenomena such as swelling of the brain, loss of consciousness, etc. Because the prostate and its accessory glands are among the organs of the body least known to laymen, this handbook will first describe their structure and function and then present the significant fact that, in the opinion of Dr. Bircher-Benner, this dreaded disease of man can be prevented by a complete vegetable diet and, in its initial stages, can be completely cured without surgery.

Since this disease enlarges the prostate as a result of noncancerous cellular proliferation, this book will also deal with cancerous hypertrophy of the prostate in order to instruct the reader in the essential differences between these two diseases.

Symptoms of inflammation can occur in the prostate for various reasons without simultaneous glandular hypertrophy, e.g. in young men. For purposes of distinction, aspects of prostatic inflammation (prostatitis) will also be explained. The instructions given in this handbook should in no way create the impression that medical examination in problems of micturition is superfluous. Without exception, in all cases of disturbances of the urinary organs, medical examination is essential to clarify their cause. Since prostatic hypertrophy occurs only in the second half of a man's life, the instructions presented here for better nutrition and health are at the same time a guide to a healthy way of life, for men as well as for women.

–Heinrich Herget, M.D.

Preface

Contents

I. Introduction

THE NATURE OF BENIGN PROSTATIC HYPERTROPHY (PROSTATISM)

In this disease nodular proliferations of the connective-tissue fibers, the smooth muscle fibers and glandular ducts of three glandular groups within the sphincter-like annulus of the prostate encircle the urethra at its outlet from the bladder. Initially, as small proliferating enlargements, they impede the elimination of urine from the bladder, but with continued enlargement of these nodular proliferations they completely block the urinary tract. The prostate does not itself form cellular proliferations, but rather it is invaded by cellular proliferations of the three glandular groups from the connective tissue mantle (urethral mantle) of the urogenital ducts. These three glandular groups discharge into the urogenital ducts very close to the numerous orifices of the prostate and both ejaculatory ducts leading from the seminal vesicles to the testes, that is, in the region of the so-called seminal colliculus of the urogenital ducts. As this cellular proliferation advances, the cells of the prostate are damaged by its pressure and pushed against the thin connective-tissue layer of the capsule encircling the prostate. Since this cellular proliferation resembles the goiter-forming proliferation of the thyroid, this disease has also been called goiter of the neck of the bladder or adenoma of the neck of the bladder, i.e. glandular hypertrophy on that part of the urethral canal which is surrounded by the prostate at the neck of the bladder. The term, prostatic hypertrophy (enlargement of the prostate), although actually inappropriate, is nevertheless generally accepted. The healthy prostate has the size and shape of a chestnut; as a result of cellular proliferation it can attain the size of a small apple, a hen's egg or even a fist.

THE CAUSE OF PROSTATIC HYPERTROPHY

This disease of cellular proliferation is caused by an increasing lack of sexual hormones. In western countries, as opposed to China and Japan where this disease occurs very infrequently, hormonal decrease becomes noticeable in men about 40 years of age and worsens in those above 50 years of age. Prostatim never afflicts young men, but affects 40-60% of men between the ages of 40 and 50 years and 60-90% of men beyond 60 years of age.

The prostate is essential for masculine procreative capacity. The prostate matures during the years of a boy's adolescence along with the maturation of the testes (gonads). During this developmental period the gonadotrophic hormones of the anterior pituitary activate the production of the sex hormone, testosterone, in the interstitial cells of Leydig, located in the heretofore dormant testes; they also cause maturation of the sperm cells (spermatozoa) from the primitive germ cells in the seminiferous tubules of both testes. Simultaneous with spermatogenesis, processes in the prostate also matures. Testosterone from the interstitial Leydig cells of the testes stimulates the growth of the prostate and both seminal vesicles. In early castration (eunuchs) the prostate does not mature. The sexually mature prostate forms within its glandular ducts the so-called prostatic secretion which has a thin, milky appearance and is weakly alkaline (basic). During the sexual process this fluid is added to the viscous semen from the testes and seminal vesicles; the latter also add fructose for the sperm cells as they leave the seminal colliculus. The sperm cells, thus gain motility from the watery prostatic secretion. The semen, too, is propelled forward by the pressure wave from the smooth and striated muscle fibers of the prostate which, during intercourse, prevents the urethra from passing urine from the bladder. Sterility results from a malfunctioning prostate, since the prostatic secretion is essential for the mobility of the sperm cells.

But in all living creatures, nature endeavors to propagate the species. Consequently, when procreative capacity is threatened, she tries to meet this emergency by utilizing equivalent organs. In many men, with today's Western way of life, procreative capacity declines after 40 years of age. Fewer sperm cells mature in the seminiferous tubules, while the glandular activity of the prostate is diminished; as a result of lower testosterone levels male libido declines as well. After age 50, these symptoms intensify in most Western men. In many women, smooth muscle fibers proliferate in the uterus, and muscle tumors (myomas) form during the time when procreative capacity is threatened due to diminishing hormone production of the ovaries, between age 36 (pre-climacteric) and age 55 climacteric. About 84% of myoma patients who require treatment are between 36 and 55 years of age. Likewise in many men, cells from the three sexual glands which encircle the prostate at the seminal colliculus proliferate in the mantle of the urethra as a result of diminished functional capacity of the male reproductive glands and push nodular proliferations into the prostate. The gynecologist Sellheim described the process of muscle cell proliferation which occurs in the muscle cells of the uterus when the functional capacity of the female reproductive glands declines as follows: "The uterus runs to weed instead of bearing fruit."

Other diseases can also have abnormal and imperfect cellular reparative effects in the human body, e.g., pernicious anemia. In that case, a lack of the blood corpuscle maturation factor, hemamine (hemopoetin from the gastric mucosa and Vitamin B_{12}) hinders the maturation of red blood cells in red bone marrow, while the liver makes an incomplete attempt to form these cells, as it does, routinely, from the second to seventh months of development of the embryo in the uterus. A similar makeshift attempt at incomplete cellular proliferation occurs in the thyroid from iodine deficiency which results in goiter formation (especially in the Alps).

Extensive proof that prostatic hypertrophy does not occur in the presence of sufficient male sexual hormone, testosterone, is provided by the Chinese and Japanese people. These people are essentially vegetarians, eating large amounts of rice. Rice, as all other types of grain, is rich in sexually active substances–vegetable sexual hormone. The soy bean, another food of the Eastern peoples, as a seed is rich in vegetable sexual hormones. All in all, the essentially vegetarian foods of the Chinese are much richer in sexually active substances than the meat- and sugar-rich diets of today's Western peoples. After the 40th year of life and especially after age 50, and with a diet lacking in vegetable sexual hormones, it obviously becomes more and more difficult for the male organism to synthesize the male sexual hormone, testosterone, from a fatty meat diet abundantly rich in cholesterol. Thus, it is clear why European and American physicians who have worked in China found that prostatic hypertrophy occurs only rarely in that country. It is also significant that the Chinese, through continuous fertile propagation and a consequent abundance of children, have attained a population of over 700 million people, the largest population of all the peoples of the world!

Further evidence that prostatic hypertrophy is caused by a lack of sexually active substances is the fact that in animals prostatic hypertrophy only occurs from a lack of sexually active substances in the food. According to the observations of veterinarians, prostatic hypertrophy occurs mostly in dogs; conspicuously in dogs living in urban households, who are often fed the food of their owners. This includes cooked and roasted meats and white flour products and sugar-rich "tidbits." Thus, they are overfed with a diet particularly poor in sexually active substances, which causes many dogs to become obese. According to the findings of veterinarians, prostatic hypertrophy seldom occurs in bulls! The latter have a diet primarily of green fodder and oats which is rich in sexually active substances. According to the findings of veterinarians and farmers, old bulls become infertile when their hay is not supplemented with enough oats, i.e., a grain diet rich in the germinative substance of the oat seedling. It is equally significant that, according to these observations, prostatic hypertrophy never occurs in stallions whose main diet from youth to old age consists of the germinative-rich substance of unhusked, unprocessed, whole-grain oats.

In eunuchs, e.g. in men who have lost their testes before sexual development, prostatic hypertrophy never occurs. This is due to the fact that in early castrati the reproductive glands behind the urethra, in the region of the seminal colliculus, do not develop due to the complete lack of testosterone. In men without testes the urethra never becomes a genital duct but functions only as a urethra, as it has since childhood. Even after 40 years of age, their reproductive glands in the region of the seminal colliculus do not change, since these glands have remained undeveloped since childhood.

PROBLEMS OF MICTURITION AS A RESULT OF PROSTATIC HYPERTROPHY

Hypertrophy of the right and left glandular groups proliferating into the prostate bilaterally at the seminal colliculus, and of the fibrous tissue in the urethral mantle at this site, causes the prostate to form two lateral lobes. This causes part of the urethral tract leading out of the bladder to become stretched lengthwise and narrowed, and the floor of the bladder to be raised. As hypertrophy progresses, the lateral lobes project into the bladder lumen and are pressed together under the internal pressure of the bladder as it fills with urine; thus, the bladder outlet becomes constricted. This occurs even more frequently when the middle glandular group, in particular, proliferates into the prostate, so that this growth projects deep into the bladder, thereby bending the portion of the urethra nearest the bladder. Under pressure of the filling bladder, a proliferating nodule of this type can form a valvelike closure of the outlet to the urethra similar to a plug. The physician can feel this enlargement of the prostate resulting from cellular proliferation by way of the rectum which adjoins the prostate.

Severe cramps associated with constriction of the bladder sometimes occur at drinking parties, when a man, who until then had only mild difficulties in micturition, suddenly can no longer urinate. With his bladder overextended from drinking, and the unfavorable cooling of his stomach with cold beer, as well as the unfavorable effect of alcohol, he suffers the pains of complete cystoplegia. The physician who is hastily called in must relieve him of this unbearable urinary overload by pushing a rubber tube (catheter) through the urethra into the bladder. This example illustrates that many men have a slight to moderate glandular hypertrophy at the neck of the bladder even when they may not have had any special problems in emptying their bladders.

However, with excessive beer drinking, the corresponding alcohol consumption, and a cooling of the stomach, several unfavorable circumstances come together. The muscle responsible for emptying the bladder (detrusor muscle) can no longer equalize the pressure of hypertrophy of the neck of the bladder, and the engorged urine no longer has an exit through the urethra. This makes the individual suddenly aware of a gradually threatening affliction which had been slowly developing. About 80% of men over 60 years of age (in Western countries) have some degree of cellular proliferation at the neck of the bladder; of these, about half have little or no appreciable difficulties in micturition until the end of their lives (in Germany today's life expectancy of men is 67 years). Thus, despite slight or moderate prostatic hypertrophy the detrusor muscle retains its functional capacity because of favorable general conditions in the abdominal cavity and in the urinary composition.

A diet rich in meat is unfavorable, because, among other things, more uric acid (from purine of the nucleic acids of the cellular nuclei of meat) must be eliminated in the urine. Diets rich in meat usually contain an excess of salt ($NaCl$), which is unfavorable because excess salt produces thirst which, in turn, leads to excess fluid intake and large quantities of urine. Besides the beer, mentioned above, and other alcohol, carbonated, alcohol-caffeine and coca-containing beverages are dangerous to the urinary bladder because of their various stimulatory effects, as are today's popular warm sweetened drinks containing purine (caffeine in bean coffee and black tea; theobromine in cocoa). The functional capacity of the urinary bladder can become even more unfavorable due to constipation with consequent narrowing of the pelvic cavity from overfilling the large intestine with feces and gas. Other impediments stem from fatty degeneration of the blood vessels (arteriosclerosis) with diminished function of the autonomic innervation of the abdominal organs; from general adiposity of the body and widespread effects of chills, especially in the abdomen and cold emanating from the feet. A lack of adequate body warmth in the region of the bladder can cause narrowing of the blood vessels of the bladder and the detrusor muscle and thereby impede its function, thus intensifying the effects of hypertrophy of the neck of the bladder. Conditions for urination also become unfavorable as a consequence of excess body heat. In overheated rooms, with heat retention in the lower abdomen from warm upholstery, the blood vessels in the region of the urinary bladder are relaxed by heat. This relaxation of the blood vessels diminishes the functional capacity of the detrusor muscle in the same way as constriction through cold. Both conditions promote over-filling and obstruction of the bladder due to cellular proliferation in the neck of the bladder.

CONSEQUENCES OF IMPAIRED MICTURITION AS A RESULT OF PROSTATIC HYPERTROPHY

The individual first becomes aware of his problem in micturition when there is no urine flow in the presence of a distinct need to urinate. The bladder finally empties itself by straining the detrusor muscle, but urine flow is feeble rather than heavy. When the detrusor muscle can no longer completely empty the bladder because of excessive constriction of the bladder neck by the hypertrophied prostate, urine remains in the bladder. The constant amount of urine which thereby remains unnaturally in the bladder causes the danger of an inflammation of the bladder mucosa due to proliferation of fission fungi (bacteria, bacilli) in the residual urine and the resulting danger of extension of inflammation to adjacent urinary passages. The residual urine remaining in the bladder also causes urine to crystallize more readily and form urinary caliculi (uric acid, phosphoric acid, oxalic acid); stones the size of grains of sand can obstruct the urethra during partial bladder evacuation.

The concerned individual tries to compensate for the limited bladder evacuation by frequent micturition (Pollackisuria), especially as the pressure-irritated bladder continually requires this. During sleep the augmented drive to urinate is especially unpleasant because sleep is disturbed and interrupted. Since the bladder sphincter muscle can be overgrown by the hypertrophic gland, it becomes leaky, and an exceedingly disagreeable trickling of urine results, with wetting of clothes and odors. The drops of urine which are discharged, sometimes by great pressure from the overfilled bladder, will moisten the inside of the upper thigh (so-called overflowing bladder; Ischuria paradoxa). The bladder tries to overcome these difficulties in micturition by strengthening its muscle layer (so-called fasciculated bladder), and to expel the urine by muscular strength. Overextension of the overfilled bladder produces intolerable distention, pains and cramps. Intensive pressing in order to evacuate the bladder can rupture blood vessels (veins), which extend over the proliferating nodules of the prostate, and thereby produce severe blood loss (hematuria). The overfilled bladder can be felt in the abdominal cavity up to the navel and can sometimes contain several liters of urine. It can create terrible stomach pains that sometimes suggest intestinal paralysis, intestinal occlusion (ileus) or even stomach cancer. Regurgitation of urine from the bladder into the ureters affects their mucosa, smooth muscle fibers and nerves. As the condition becomes advanced, the urinary regurgitation extends from both ureters into both renal pelvises, and, as the latter come to contain excessive amount of urine, crystallization occurs, tending to form kidney stones. The urine regurgitated into the renal pelvis exerts severe pressure on the glomerulus and tubules; this can adversely affect the urine-forming capability of the kidneys. The kidneys excrete a urine so dilute and watery that abnormal loss of water and potassium from the body tissues occurs along with elevated residual nitrogen levels in the blood. Gradually, uremia develops, as substances normally secreted into the urine from the blood are retained. Acidosis of the blood with azotemia results. Warning symptoms of uremia are loss of appetite, bad breath, constipation, unusual fatigue, general depression, as well as an obvious loss of memory resulting from toxic effects on nerve cells of the cerebral cortex, and an agonizing thirst. In this condition the organism tries to eliminate nitrogenous wastes through the stomach and intestines instead of the kidneys, which produces vomiting and diarrhea along with weight loss. If these warning symptoms of the onset of uremia are not completely relieved, progressive uremia will also affect the heart and circulation, the pulse accelerates and blood pressure falls;

cerebral edema produces drowsiness and finally unconsciousness and fatal lesions.

THE TREATMENT OF PROSTATIC HYPERTROPHY

If a man in his forties notices the onset of even a slight problem in micturition, e.g. a decrease in urine flow, he should consult a physician or a urologist. If the physician confirms an incipient prostatic hypertrophy, the individual must immediately alter (a) his diet and (b) his general mode of life, in order to avoid the gradual worsening of pains in micturition and its usual consequences. A vegetable diet rich in sexually active substances will suppress further prostatic hypertrophy. Defecation at least twice daily will prevent constipation and flatulence in the intestine. Furthermore, a healthy vegetable diet without alcohol, and supplemented with milk and dairy products and sufficient daily muscular exercise is necessary, to improve general metabolism and circulation and to prevent fatty degeneration of blood vessels and deficiency in heat production. This diet and total way of life must be strictly and permanently adhered to, so that all problems of micturition will disappear. If one reverts to the incorrect diet and habits of today's usual Western way of life, under the pressures of an automated society, then the danger of difficulties in micturition reappear and, according to age, may be more profound.

The following is an example of permanently successful treatment with a diet rich in sexually active substances and a regulated way of life:

"A 54-year-old professor had experienced disagreeable problems with micturition for some time. The need to urinate had become noticeably more frequent, while the amount of urine eliminated each time was less than before. Since he continued to have increasing need to urinate, but, upon rushing to the toilet, would always have to wait some time before urine began to flow, he consulted a physician. The doctor diagnosed prostatic hypertrophy and told him that an operation of the hypertrophied gland was necessary. However, the patient wanted above all to avoid surgical intervention and, thus, sought my advice. Examination by way of the rectum revealed enlargement of the prostate to about the size of a small apple. I explained to the patient that it was altogether possible that he could be freed of his complaints without an operation if he would follow a regulated way of life with a fundamentally correct diet. The necessity of complete body warmth and of totally avoiding cold or partially warm feet, knees, buttocks, loins, and stomach was also pointed out. Like most of today's Western people, he suffered from cold feet and intestinal weakness.

The patient carefully followed the prescribed way of life and converted to a high-value diet, emphasizing fresh foods. Bircher-Benner's *Fruit and Raw Vegetable Dishes* served as a guide. He learned to appreciate the benefits of applying water of alternating temperatures which increases blood flow and maintains the temperature of the lower half of the body. (Baths of the lower legs up to the knees, starting warm, increasing to hot, then cooling off with cold water, and alternating this pattern frequently; sitz-baths in which only the buttocks and abdomen are submerged in the changing bath water; and baths in which the entire lower half of the body is submerged in the changing bath water.)

With all these measures came a gradual establishment of orderly conditions in the large intestine—with disappearance of flatulence and constipation there was no longer spatially constrictive pressure on the adjacent bladder organs; temperature equilibrium, no more interference with the prostate and the resulting relief from disabilities have now been maintained for 8 years.

Cystoplegia is remedied by the physician by catheterization of the bladder. Catheterization is, occasionally, so beneficial that the deceptive hope may arise that prostatic hypertrophy can be permanently compensated by self-catheterization, or by a permanently implanted catheter. This creates increased danger of inflammation of the urinary passages and fungal transmission, as hypertrophy of the prostrate progresses.

If the patient delays seeking treatment and the residual urine content of the bladder is over 100 cc., hypertrophy must be remedied surgically to avoid the danger of progressive uremia; and the loss of sexual reproductive capacity must be taken in one's stride. Surgical treatment involves extirpation of the nodular proliferation which encapsulates the prostate (prostatectomy); this means entering either above the urinary bladder or from the perineum or from the rectum. Insofar as this frees the prostate from the pressure of nodular proliferation, it can recover and again form the prostatic secretion. Reproductive function is, however, lost because the operation causes the internal sphincter muscle of the urinary bladder to leak, so that, during the sexual process, semen flows into the bladder and is not ejaculated through the urogenital duct. If surgical extirpation is performed from the perineum (between the anus and the external genitalia) the nerves which mediate sexual desires, are often injured, and erection during sexual intercourse becomes impossible. Electrosection over the ureters removes the nodular proliferation of the prostate by operative diathermy. This also causes the internal sphincter muscle of the neck of the bladder to become leaky so that semen goes into the bladder; reproductive capacity is, thus, again impaired.

THE PREVENTION OF PROSTATIC HYPERTROPHY WITH FOODS RICH IN SEXUALLY ACTIVE SUBSTANCES

Sexually active substances, sexual hormones, are as essential to plants as they are to man and animal. Every Fall man sees the hazelnut tree forming male pollen, and in Spring this is generously spread around (plant semen). Thus, in early Spring the female blossoms which have appeared can be fertilized. Male and female sexual hormone are necessary for the hazelnut tree to form male and female blossoms. They are also necessary for all flowers, vegetable-fruits, and fruit trees whose white, pink and red blossoming splendor delights us every Spring. Biochemical research, e.g. by Loewe at the University of Dorpat, demonstrated the male sexual hormone, androkinin, in male willow and birch catkin and in yeast. Already by 1927, the researchers Loewe, Lange and Spoke, at the University of Dorpat, had found the female sexual hormone, thelykinin, in female willow blossoms. In 1933, Professors Butenandt and Jakobi of Gottingen prepared 18 mg female hormone in crystalline form from 50 kg palm seed husks. In animal experiments, this substance produced the same estrus actions on the vaginal mucosa of female mice as crystalline estradiol (the present name for follicular hormone) which is found, for example, in the urine of pregnant women or pregnant mares. Sexually active substances from man or animal can also reverse the process in afflicted trees which heretofore had not blossomed, to cause them to blossom and bear fruit, by fertilizing them with urine from pregnant women or pregnant cows or sheep, etc.

Man and animals can form sexually active substances from steroids which occur in plant organisms as well as in the organism of man and animal. However, for man as for animals it is evidently more efficient to administer sexually active substances in food. This is apparent in the illnesses associated with the climacteric in men and women, where administration of food rich in sexually active substances proves beneficial when diets low in such substances had previously been followed. The same is true for animals where, for example, conditions in the aging bull show that prostatic hypertrophy and sexual incapacity can occur if its hay fodder (which is low in such substances) does not contain an added oat diet rich in germinative substances. Researchers, such as M. Dohrn, Poll, Blotevogel, O. O. Fellner, H. Much, and others, investigated the occurrence of sexually active substances in segments of plants and found that all bulbous vegetables, especially celery root, are rich in sexually active substances, as are seasoning herbs (parsley, chives, chervil, etc.), and wild herbs (e.g. dandelion, whose green leaves are edible as salad and whose yellow blossoms are also edible). Researchers, such as J. Vague, F. Grandel, and others, also investigated plant and animal fats for their content of sexually active substances and showed the superiority of vegetable fats with respect to their content of the sex hormone, estrogen, over that of animal fats. Thus, 1 kg of cold-pressed olive oil contains 400 units of estrogen, compared to 10 units in 1 kg pork fat. Very high estrogen content is found in palm, soya bean, peanut and linseed oils; especially high estrogen levels are found in cereal germ (e.g., 2000 units/kg in wheat germ) and in the oil pressed from cereal germ, namely wheat germ oil, 1000/kg; rice germ oil, 4000/kg; corn seed oil, 6000/kg. Wood nettle seeds, which were used in ancient folklore, for the treatment of male and female infertility, long before the discovery of sexually active substances, contain 14,000 units/kg.

Aside from the aforementioned nutrients, edible vegetable seeds, especially in their germ, are very rich in sexually active substances. These include wheat grain, which is edible as cracked wheat (pre-soaked in water), wheat germ, whole-wheat flour and its products, such as whole-wheat bread, whole-wheat cakes, whole-wheat dumplings, and other whole-grain products made from rye, oats (germ containing oat flakes!), millet, rice (brown, unpolished rice), corn, barley (the chief grain of the Hunza, who are sexually fertile until very late in life); similarly seeds, such as hazelnuts, walnuts, pine nuts, linseed, sunflower seeds, Brazil nuts, sweet almonds, pumpkin seeds, edible chestnuts, coconuts, young peas (sweet and fresh from the pod), caraway; in addition, all other vegetable-fruits such as tomatoes, bell peppers, cucumbers and pumpkins. Especially included amongst the fruits are berries (strawberries, raspberries, blackberries, red currants, gooseberries, blueberries); grapes, apples and pears, because in all of these, their stones, which are their seeds, are edible. Additionally, cauliflower and artichokes (both of which are flower heads) are also rich in germinative active substances. Adherence to this type of diet, with its abundant supply of germinative substances for the organism, not only has a preventive effect with respect to prostatic hypertrophy, but also has, in the early stages of prostatic hypertrophy, a so-called anabolic effect on the blood vessels in the proliferation at the neck of the bladder and the adjacent organs which have been irritated by difficulties in micturition. Thus, the bladder, urethra, and the internal and external sphincter muscles of the bladder are strengthened, and the inflammatory blood congestion in these organs, produced by difficulties in micturition, is counteracted. Similar results have been observed by urologists after injection of sex hormones (estrogen–androgen). Reduction of this inflammatory blood congestion improves the function of the detrusor muscle and of the bladder sphincter muscles, even in already existing prostatic hypertrophy.

The best possible type of diet for the whole human organism, for nerve cells, heart and blood vessels, viscera, glands, skin and bones, is one which provides vegetable foods rich in sexually active compounds which in their natural and fresh state contain high energy substances. It is a diet with abundant natural vegetable protein (not heated protein), enzymes and vitamins, minerals with an excess of base and trace elements, sugar substances and a balanced mixture of saturated and unsaturated fatty acids. Its comprehensive effect is important for the gradual amelioration of all disturbances in micturition resulting from prostatic hypertrophy, since the better the condition and function of the whole organism, the more favorable the effects on the urinary organs. A strong and healthy process of nerve conduction in the whole organism produces favorable neural effects on the urinary organs. Freedom from cardiac and circulatory disorders also produces a favorable effect on the blood circulation of the urinary organs. The better the condition of the mucosa of the digestive and respiratory tracts from high potency foods, the better the results for the urinary organs. Greater functional capacity of a strong and healthy skin, means greater capacity to aid the urinary organs in the necessary elimination of metabolic end products. The usual diet of Western man frequently produces difficulties in micturition due to prostatic hypertrophy. This diet, aside from its low content of sexually active substances, is unhealthy for the urinary organs because of its high content of meat which burdens the urinary organs with the elimination of excess uric acid from purine in the nucleic acid of the cell nuclei in any slaughter house food, even organ meats and fish. The purine content of young, white meat is greater than that of meat from older animals. Aside from this, constipation favors the formation of indolę (similar to skatole), which is highly toxic to metabolism and nerve cells; it is formed from the amino acid, tryptophan (abundant in meats), due to a lack of lactic acid in the lower ileum (much indican is eliminated in the urine). Fatty meat, in the form of highly fatty roasts of force-fed goose, duck, chicken, turkey, fattened pig and fattened oxen, additionally contributes to the troublesome effect of meat protein in our highly sedentary society. The most widespread illness in Western people is fatty degeneration of the inner wall of the arteries from fatty cholesterol and food rich in saturated fatty acids (bacon, pork sausage, ham, pork and goose fat). These are the chief causes of heart ailments from coronary vessel damage, blood pressure problems, damage to the arteries of the limbs, propensity for strokes, arterial thromboses and embolisms. Such diseases and functional deficiencies naturally have additional unfavorable effects on the difficulties of micturition from prostatic hypertrophy. In meat diets, the excessive use of the mineral compound cooking salt (sodium chloride) also has adverse effects on kidneys and the metabolic processes of the entire body.

Similarly unfavorable is modern man's diet of refined flour, and intake of excessive white sugar (in and on pastries, beverages, candies, chocolate, canned fruits, preserves, spirits and liquors). White flour products are low in vitamins because the husks of wheat and corn grains have been removed in the mill. They are especially low in Vitamin B_1, and are low in lime and mineral substances, because the minerals of cereal grains occur primarily in the husks. Even more unfavorable than white flour is the abundant ingestion of white sugar. It is completely without mineral substances, vitamins (except for a small amount of B_2 riboflavin), albumin and fats, in contrast to the variety of nutrients in the sweet beet from which white sugar is obtained by heating and refining processes. Abundant ingestion of white flour foods and white sugar causes the deposition of fat in the body with the conversion of its excessively large amounts of carbohydrates into stored fat since there is no other way in which the body can utilize the excessively large quantities of carbohydrates. This carbohydrate diet contributes to today's unusually widespread adiposity and obesity, diabetes, weakness toward fungal and viral germs (influenza, virus among others), and pus-forming strepto- and staphylococci, liver disease, damaged nerve cells, and the desire for addictive and pep drugs (nicotine in tobacco, alcohol, opium, morphine, hashish-marijuana, cocaine) and the so-called arousal amines (like pervitin, etc.) all of which exacerbate the problem of micturition in prostatic hypertrophy.

All of the above mentioned foods, which predominate in today's Western nutrition together with boiled, over-salted potatoes and vegetables from which the minerals and vitamins contained in the cooking juices have been poured off, offer diminished energy and thus, diminished effectiveness. In contrast to these modern foods, a high potency vegetable diet in the form of uncooked vegetables was proposed by Dr. M. Bircher-Benner in 1895 and was used by him as the basis for treating the sick in his institute of "Kinetic Energy" (today: Bircher-Benner Clinic in Zurich) with remarkable success in treating the most varied diseases.

Uncooked vegetarian foods provide nutrition on the highest level of energy and of greatest potential, because, in their natural state, they are the building blocks of cells.

Moreover, this diet has not been harmed (sterilized) by the heating processes of cooking, roasting, baking, stewing, braising, steaming or dehydrating, melting, frying, oxidation, infrared and short-wave irradiation. The natural, fresh state of the cells of uncooked vegetarian food provides man with protein at its full energy level. These foods also contain their entire original content of enzymes, vitamins, minerals and trace elements.

In practice this means that today's typical breakfast which consists of sweetened coffee or cocoa, white toast, marmalade and often also a soft boiled egg, is substituted by fresh fruit according to season, e.g. in Bircher-Muesli (see Recipes) and, on cool days, a warm drink of rose hip or herb tea such as peppermint, yarrow, etc., sweetened with honey or fruit juice. For the first days, whole-grain bread should be omitted, later whole-grain bread is allowed and, according to preference, some fresh butter or vegetable margarine, also a cup of milk, according to need and hunger.

The modern-day lunch* consists of meat soup, cooked or roasted meat with white flour dumplings or overcooked potatoes, white flour pudding or compote or sweet pastry, with or without alcoholic beverage or a cup of black coffee. This is replaced for the first 3 to 5 days of treatment with fresh salad of vegetables according to season, including leaf, tuber and fruit-vegetables (tomatoes, red and green peppers, etc.), prepared with lemon juice and cold-pressed oil, without cooking salt; nuts can be added if very hungry. On the 4th or 5th day after start of treatment, some whole-grain bread or unpeeled, steamed potatoes can be added if desired; for lunch on cool days, supplement this by some warm water with tasty, fresh vegetable juice or with vegetable broth (no cooking salt and meat extract), seasoned with some sea salt or herb salt. After another 3 to 5 days of pure raw foods, vegetable soup or whole-grain soup can be consumed; also whole-wheat flour dumplings with herb sauce and, if very hungry, whole-wheat pastry (e.g., cherry cake or similar fruit cakes). Fruit juice is best as a table drink. Dinner is similar to breakfast and lunch, but less extensive.

---

* In Germany the main meal is eaten at lunch.—Ed.

After 3 to 5 days of only raw foods, adding, on one day, whole-grain bread or potatoes, one will appreciate the advantages of this carefully conceived diet for its special curative effects. The functional strength of the digestive organs is increased by this easily digested enzyme-rich diet. It supplies the vitamins required to overcome the existing lack in vitamin supply. The body's reserve of basic mineral substances will be augmented, thereby aiding the alkaline reserve of the blood. For a permanent diet, the regular consumption of whole-grain baked goods (whole-grain bread, whole-wheat rolls, whole-wheat cake, etc.), boiled or baked potatoes and vegetables, as well as whole-grain soups, vegetable sausage made from soy beans, pressed yeast juice, etc., are recommended after and along with the raw foods, because these foods are especially convenient, vary the menu and are available throughout the year. The proportion of raw foods to carefully prepared hot vegetable foods, including milk, in the permanent diet should be about half and half. But each meal, breakfast too, should be started with the noblest and most valuable food, fresh fruit and fresh vegetables. To satisfy the need of the body for heat in sedentary people, a hot water bottle can be placed on the body at meal time (abdomen, feet, upper thigh, small of the back) for complete warmth; after the first bite of raw food, plenty of warm liquids of the type described above, can be drunk.

The amount of food consumed at a meal will vary according to the requirements of the body. One should not eat without and above hunger! Over-eating does not invigorate but rather weakens the digestive organs as well as the heart and blood vessels; nor does it lengthen life, but rather shortens it and is detrimental to the beauty of the human body. Countless people, both young and old, today in Western countries are overweight since it has become a customary right, we tend to accept it as normal, though it should be considered a serious mistake. According to surveys by life insurance companies of millions and millions of people, the greatest life expectancy occurs in those who are thin; the so-called industrialized nations already have a considerably lower life expectancy; the life expectancy is lowest in the obese, with their hamster-like cheeks, fat necks, double chins, fat rounded backs and pot-bellies.

A comprehensive vegetarian diet, as described above, with or without milk and dairy products according to taste, guarantees man the best possible supply of protein (protein of fresh living green leaf vegetables, of quiescent as well as growing wheat seedlings and of nuts is especially valuable). This has been proven by extensive medical observations, as well as by scientifically regulated diets, e.g. by Prof. Lintzell (Germany), Prof. Hegsted (USA), Prof. Kuratsune (Japan), which confirm earlier investigations, e.g. by Prof. Hindhede (Denmark), Prof. McCollum (USA). That the protein in a complete vegetable diet is not sufficient for man is a current and frequently held, erroneous, pseudoscientific assertion. In our time, the enormous spread of high blood pressure disease—men, too with prostatic hypertrophy often have elevated blood pressure—occurs when the protein requirements are not met with vegetable protein which has the advantage of being able to lower blood pressure, but with animal protein, especially meats, which raise blood pressure, as was clearly demonstrated by the extensive investigation of Profs. Mayer and Gutzeit in Breslaw in 1944.

At the start of the diet, everybody first loses some weight, even those who tend to be too thin, because much of the food previously eaten had deposited salt in the body which was not adequately excreted by the kidneys, leading to water retention in the body cells. Since uncooked vegetarian foods are eaten without the addition of salt, the kidneys succeed in eliminating the stored salt, via the urine. After this reduction in salt and water thin people slowly gain weight with this high potency food. In contrast, obese people slowly lose fat. It is urgently advised not to tell one's friends about the change in diet until healthful results are clearly evident; talking about it at the start of treatment, increases the difficulties because most people are not knowledgeable about it, living as everybody else does and therefore, instinctively slandering the diet.

With this diet, the capacity to form sperm in the testes is considerably increased in men; and 50-year-old men, in whom sexual capability had already entirely or almost entirely disappeared, to their surprise, can experience a remarkable return to the sexual capacity of their youth.

People with inflammation of the gastric mucosa, gastric hyperacidity, gastric or duodenal ulcers, liver ailments, or gall bladder irritations may experience unpleasant problems with the digestive mucosa in metabolizing the acids in fresh fruits (apple acid, grape acid, citric acid). It is usually recommended to destroy the fruit acids, which are so valuable for the healthy individual, by cooking the fruit; however, this robs the individual of the value of fresh fruit. We recommend that the fruit acids of fresh fruits be neutralized by Muesli, with pre-soaked oat flakes, milk and nut purée. It is also possible to neutralize the fruit acids by eating fruit together with a gruel of agar-agar (dried algae) cream of rice, oats, barley or linseed, or almond milk; pressed fruit juice can be mixed with creamed cereals to neutralize acids. Freshly prepared pressed potato juice and pressed savoy cabbage juice are particularly efficacious for sensitive digestive mucosa. Highly sensitive people must avoid citrus fruits for a prescribed length of time. For further advice, consult the *Bircher-Benner Nutrition Plan for Digestive Problems,* and the *Bircher-Benner Nutrition Plan for Liver and Gallbladder Problems.*

Inflammation of the urinary passages in prostatic hypertrophy can also be influenced by fungal toxins, by infected root canals and gums, by irritated tonsils, an inflamed gallbladder, and by phlebitis. Such focal toxins also diminish the therapeutic effects of uncooked vegetarian food. If necessary, the infected teeth must be pulled. (For details on strengthening and detoxifying the tonsils refer to my exposé in "Reform-Rundshau," 1962/1.) Concerning phlebitis and also hemorrhoids, which through inflammatory symptoms can increase the irritation of the urinary passages in the region of the prostate, refer to handbook, vol. 12 for venous diseases (Bircher-Benner Publication).

Difficulties in micturition may occur without prostatic hypertrophy from paralytic symptoms of the urinary bladder as a result of multiple sclerosis. Sometimes prostatic hypertrophy occurs in the presence of multiple sclerosis. Information concerning this disease can be found in the handbook for people with multiple sclerosis (Bircher-Benner Publication, vol. 11).

Intestinal constipation severely constricts space in the abdomen and, thus, burdens the urinary passages. Some people have an intestinal evacuation only once every 2 days, some only once every 3 or 4 days. Many people consume 2 large snacks between the basic 3 meals. People who have an intestinal evacuation once every 2 days, thus, retain remnants of 6-10 meals in the large intestine. This is an immense amount, consisting, because of our modern diet, mainly of meat residue which forms foul smelling gases as a result of protein decomposition. The longer the digestive remnants remain in the large intestine, the greater the increase in fission fungi from the decay process; gases will therefore fill the intestine and exert a constrictive pressure on the other abdominal organs, including the bladder, the neck of the bladder and its sphincter muscles, thereby causing additional difficulties in prostatic hypertrophy. The chief cause of constipation of the intestine, which empties itself automatically in healthy individuals on a daily basis almost as often as food is consumed (thus, on the average of thrice with three meals per day), is today's customary incorrect diet and sedentary way of life. For this reason, a high-potency diet rich in natural vegetable foods, and sufficient bodily activity, especially walking and proper breathing are the most important therapeutic measures against constipation. The effect of a diet rich in uncooked vegetable foods on the functional capacity of the intestine is explained by the improved total functional capacity of the millions of small blood vessels (capillaries) of the intestinal mucosa, the intestinal glands, the autonomic nerves and the smooth muscle fibers of the vessels supplying the intestine (capillary research of Prof. Gansslen, research on the permeability of small blood vessels and cell walls by Prof. Eppinger). The intestinal mucosa are supplied with vitamins in balanced proportions (e.g., the proportion of vitamins C to B_1). There is also improved mechanical stimulation of peristaltic movement of the digestive products along the intestine by the cellulose fiber content in the food (cellulose in the skin of stone-fruit and the bran in the husk of whole grains). This diet also furnishes a better intestinal environment for formation of lactic acid from the sugars in the vegetable foods–coli-fission fungi in the lower part of the ileum are prevented from forming the highly toxic indole and skatole from the protein constituent, tryptophan (research by Prof. Baumgartel)–and for acidophilic fission fungi in the small intestine and for coli-fission fungi in the large intestine. The positive effects of muscular activity, especially walking, on the intestine, are due to an improved supply to the entire body, including the intestine, with oxygen as a result of deeper respiration. The intestine, like all other organs, can, thus, better utilize nutrients by augmented cellular oxidation; moreover, deep breathing when walking causes an intensified and beneficial massaging action of the diaphragm on the intestine. Walking and running also improves venous blood flow from the legs and abdominal organs.

In most people bowel movements become regular in a surprisingly short time after conversion to a high potency diet and abundant muscular exercise. Some people may need specific foods to stimulate the bowels: damsons and figs among the stoned fruits; linseed (drinkable as tea with honey); sesame seeds amongst the oil fruits; rhubarb and spinach as vegetables (the saponins in spinach stimulate peristalsis according to Prof. Heupke); buttermilk, whey, curdled milk or natural yogurt rather than sweet milk. For some people medication with powerful acidophilic fission fungi for the small intestine and coli-fission fungi for the large intestine, is required. Constipation is also, sometimes, associated with an early suppression of the reflex urge to defecate; e.g., some suppress the urge to defecate in childhood, when it arises during play, and later on, due to erroneous social constraints, in school or in business. In order to reactivate the neural stimulus for opening the sphincter muscle of the rectum, a toilet must be found daily, morning, noon and evening at the same time and bowel movement must be awaited patiently. It may be helpful to turn on the water faucet and thus listen to the splashing noise of running water for several minutes. Some people may have psychologically conditioned intestinal cramps or sluggishness which cause constipation. These can be successfully treated, at least for a limited time, by hypnosis (Prof. Forel). The permanent effect of hypnosis on psychological problems is, however, questionable. In no case should a dependency on hypnosis be allowed to form, which would necessitate becoming dependent upon daily hypnosis, even during vacation, etc. More beneficial psychotherapy helps the individual to be involved, not passively as in hypnosis, but to cooperate in finding an appropriate mode of self influence (Coué, Prof. Brauchle) or, cooperating with the psychiatrist, to search the unconscious in ordeal to overcome inappropriate emotional responses.

In some people who are prone to chills, bowel movement can be facilitated by muscular relaxation. This can be achieved by lying down on a comfortable sofa and thoroughly warming the abdomen with a hot water bottle. During this period of relaxation, singing or music (e.g., from a record) can help to alleviate mental and nervous tension.

Finally, constipation can always be relieved with enemas of lukewarm water or, better yet, a camomile solution, with the aid of an enema apparatus with tubing (irrigator) or a large rubber ball syringe. Soap solutions should not be used. Such solutions cause leaching of the mucosa of the large intestine. The chlorinated tap water available in big cities should be boiled to bind the chlorine to the lime in the water. Such intestinal lavages are completely safe and can be carried out more than once a day to relieve cases of stomach flatulence. If the high potency diet is followed, sooner or later, such lavages will no longer be necessary. Aside from these enemas with abundant lukewarm fluid, there is still the possibility of routine introduction of cold water into the intestine by means of a small rubber bulb syringe. Refrigerated water may be used after it has been boiled to remove chlorine. The small amount of cold water thereby introduced evokes a stimulus for bowel movement which, however, can be easily suppressed, because the volume introduced is much smaller than the quantity of fluid in the previously described warm intestinal lavage. This small amount of water can be retained in the rectum (it is therefore called retention enema). Since cold water can remain in the rectum (hence, also named chronic enema) the cold stimulus will produce a powerful flow of blood into the rectal wall and thereby enhance rectal mobility. This type of enema can be carried out daily, morning, noon and evening for 2 to 4 weeks, as a kind of exercise for the large intestine.

The spread of intestinal constipation is also associated with circulatory disturbances in the stomach organs as a result of congestion of venous blood in the abdominal region from bending over during endless sitting behind a desk, on the assembly line, in the car, etc. That is why the augmented and stimulated blood flow through the abdominal organs due to bodily activity is also helpful in constipation; at the same time, the increased and accelerated arterial flow and the likewise accelerated venous flow in the abdomen are beneficial to the urinary organs. Sitzbaths and abdominal exercise also serve this purpose. For a sitzbath, one seats oneself at some convenient time of day, but never with a full stomach, in a round sitzbath tub, metal or plastic, in comfortably warm water. Feet, lower legs and lower halves of the thighs remain above water as well as the upper body. Slowly, one allows hot water to be added until the buttocks, hips, small of the back and stomach up to the lower ribs are immersed in water. The heat stimulus causes the blood vessels of the whole abdominal cavity to expand, including the digestive glands, intestine and urinary organs. At the same time, all these organs relax because the water is heavier than the air which otherwise surrounds the body. Such reduction in tissue tension is also advantageous for the circulation of all these organs. Once the skin is reddened by the heat of the hot water and the whole body feels sufficiently warm, leave the sitzbath and rinse off the middle of the body with cold water or shower until feeling refreshed. This refreshing cold stimulus also improves circulation in the abdominal organs, because the cold stimulus tightens the blood vessels so that the blood-vessel walls become more lively in carrying fresh oxygenated blood to the organs and used carbon-dioxide-laden blood away from the organs.

Similarly improved circulation for all abdominal organs is produced by exercises of the middle of the body with abdominal and hip exercise. In order to expel gases from the intestine, these exercises can also be scheduled, whenever convenient, during the normal course of the day. Standing lightly on both legs, for example, one bends the upper body vigorously, and as deeply as possible, to the left and to the right; this alternately stretches and relaxes the abdominal muscles, hip, gluteal and psoas muscles. All these muscles will also be thoroughly exercised if one lies on the back on a pad and raises the outstretched legs to an oblique position, remains with the legs in this position, and alternately raises and lowers the legs. Everyone can perform these exercises for the middle of the body while standing or lying down. For many people, the stomach muscles are today amongst the least developed muscles of the body. Many have exceptionally weak stomach muscles from overextension of the abdominal wall as a result of an extensive potbelly. All the muscles of the middle of the body are strengthened by these exercises; the muscle fibers enlarge under the stimulus and in all abdominal organs, including urinary organs and intestines; circulation is increased.

INFLAMMATION OF THE PROSTATE (PROSTATITIS)

Prostatitis is not to be confused with prostatism or prostatic hypertrophy. Like any other organ in the body, which becomes inflamed as a reaction to bacterial infection, so the prostate can swell from inflammation and become painful. This is very often the case when the gonococcus is active in gonorrhea of the urethra. In this case, the gonoccocci migrate from the urethral mucosa toward the prostate. Since in recent years the number of cases of gonorrhea has increased sharply in adolescents in Western countries–associated among other things, with the American type of social life, the party–young people of this age may already suffer from inflammation of the prostate. Such germs can also be transported to the prostate via the blood. The symptoms of an abrupt onset (acute) or, in other cases, a more lingering onset of prostatic inflammation, are pains in the region of the perineum, increasing during bowel movement and in sitting. Particularly severe cases start with high fever and shivering. All these symptoms are, therefore, entirely different from those of prostatic hypertrophy. But the prostate does enlarge, since any organ inflammation involves swelling. The swelling in prostatic inflammation is, however, very sensitive to pressure, which is confirmed by the physician as he examines from the rectum and finds that the inflamed swollen prostate is clearly hot. In the inflamed prostate, purulent flocks (abscesses) can form, from which the physician removes the pus with a suction syringe, although, sometimes, a surgical incision is required to relieve the pressure. Frequent urinary drive and retention of urine from the pressure of the swelling on the neck of the bladder also occur in this disease of the prostate, but with other, very differently associated symptoms than in prostatic hypertrophy. The treatment of prostatic inflammation should be left to the physician. Acute inflammation of the prostate can become chronic if not fully healed, and may lead to prostatic atrophy. In some men, after experiencing the disease and as it fades away, a psychic delusion concerning the prostate can arise (so-called prostatic neurosis), in which pain in the anus and in the sacral region is suggested, and the individual, still under the after-effects of the fright from the previously diseased prostate, suffers apprehension of sexual weakness and impotence.

This ailment requires treatment of body and mind.

PROSTATIC CARCINOMA

Cancer of the prostate is a malignant cellular proliferation which never emanates from the accessory sexual glands in the region of the seminal colliculus of the urethra, but always from the cells of the prostate itself, actually, mostly from the margin of the posterior lobe or the left or right lateral lobes. Since prostatic carcinoma occurs mainly after the 50th to 60th year of life, prostatic hypertrophy can occur simultaneously from the accessory glands in the region of the seminal colliculus. Difficulties in micturition also occur in this cancerous disease of the prostate. The physician, consulted because of the difficulties in micturition, upon examining the prostate from the rectum, finds totally different conditions than in the case of an adenoma of the neck of the bladder; namely, he feels an obviously hard prostate. From these results, the physician can confirm the presence of prostatic carcinoma using various additional tests for urinary diseases. The cells of the prostatic carcinoma, like the cancerous cells of other organs, derive energy from fructose, by anaerobic fermentation processes; this, in contrast to the vigorous oxygen consumption of noncancerous cells. Cancer of the prostate, when it penetrates into the soft portions of the pelvis with cancerous rests (daughter tumors), causes pain as in sciatica, sore hip. It frequently pushes cancerous proliferations into the pelvic bones and lumbar vertebrae, and, much more infrequently, into the lungs and liver. Prostatic carcinoma is a form of organ cancer, among the cancerous diseases generally which, at this time, occur most frequently as lung cancer (bronchial cancer). Presently, every 5th person dies from cancer, whereas 20 years ago, every 6th person died therefrom.

Lung cancer, which occurs noticeably were frequently wherever cigarette smoking is on the increase, should demonstrate to laymen to what extent cancer is also a condition caused by a certain way of life and the disregard for life's rules.

PREREQUISITIES FOR FITNESS AND HEALTH OF OLDER PEOPLE

Through the interplay of various circumstances–increased concern for the care of the new-born, the resulting reduction in infant mortality, widespread health insurance and the ensuing exceptional increase in medical and clinical treatment of all peoples, care of the aged, epidemic and domestic hygene–an increased life expectancy has been attained in the last century in Western countries. Unfortunately, the occurrence of disease–barring contagious and infectious diseases–has increased simultaneously, because of the tremendous increase of creeping diseases such as: fatty degeneration of the arteries (coronary vessel damage, cardiac infarction, blood flow disturbances with connective-tissue necrosis, blood clot formation, cerebral sclerosis with diminished mental and psychic function, strokes with organ impairment), rheumatism, cancer, multiple sclerosis, neuro-phychic disturbances (neurovegetative dystonia, psychoneuroses, organ neuroses). A lengthened life is thereby frequently only a life of accumulating pains.

As opposed to these regrettable circumstances, threatening not only the individual, but mankind, there are powerful possibilities for a turn for the better. The human body is built of nutritive energy and derives its work energy from nutrition. Basically sound nutrition for all peoples is indispensable for raising the health standards of peoples of all classes. The exposé on prostatic hypertrophy demonstrated the disease-producing role of nutrition low in energy foods which slowly produce damage. In this case, it is a diet which, after mechanical processing in the mill, is disastrously low in natural, sexually active substances. Today's youth should receive high energy foods, right from the start, in order to prevent diseases and damage in the so-called male and female climacteric and in old age. If this diet is followed, as prescribed in this book, with its high level of energy available in the proteins consumed as natural vegetable albumin, higher protein consumption will not be necessary in old age. Likewise, this diet eliminates the necessity to supplement one's diet with vitamins, in the form of vitamin pills, because the total diet as described here is rich in all vitamins available in vegetable foods. These foods do not always completely supply vitamin

B_{12} and vitamin D. With a way of life as prescribed herein and, if necessary, with incipient administration of suitable intestinal bacteria, very favorable conditions will develop in the human intestine for guaranteeing the provision of B_{12} in healthy intestinal flora. (It has recently been found that parsley is also rich in B_{12}.)

Vitamin D is formed in the skin of certain regions of the body from the steroids of the skin through the energizing action of the ultraviolet rays of sunlight. In large cities the ultraviolet irradiation is greatly reduced by smoke, soot and smog which layer over the city. However, by following the active mode of life prescribed in this book with daily outings, especially long outings on Sundays, by profiting from fresh air and sun on the beach, or working in the garden, even the city dweller can obtain sufficient sunlight and the necessary supply of Vitamin D. A stay in the sun is recommended, not in excess to rapidly acquire a fashionable tan, but rather according to bodily well-being, thus, for example avoiding the blazing sunlight of the hot season.

Smoking should be completely eliminated; detailed investigations have shown that it is misleading to expect only minimal damage from filter cigarettes. In women the effects of smoking on the reproductive organs is even more disasterous than in men. To completely refrain from smoking after an established smoking habit is rewarding by strengthening the personality psychically and physically.

Alcohol should also be avoided completely without exception by men and women–as a truly free personal decision. Alcohol, whether in the form of beer or fermented wine or liquor, is damaging even in small quantities, physically and mentally. Drinking does not really "heighten the spirits," but rather makes one negligent, which, as demonstrated by thorough investigation of traffic accidents, can prove disastrous in land, water or air traffic. In these times of tremendously increasing automobile traffic, alcohol usage is no longer a private matter, but a manifestation of irresponsibility toward human society and life in general. When consumed in large quantities, alcohol is very damaging to liver, heart, stomach, nerve cells and blood vessels. It also contributes considerably to fatty degeneration of the body. In these times, where man can unleash the tremendous power of atomic and nuclear fission, even a temporary reduction in mental clarity due to the effects of alcohol is of the greatest danger to all life on earth. To use alcohol for mental relaxation and as a sedative is unjustified. To relieve mental and bodily tensions with alcohol brings new tension. There are several effective means of relieving tension: comfortably stretching out on a couch, a hearty song or listening to music from a record player if one is not oneself a musician, reading a contemplative poem, best of all self searching and investigating what actually motivates one in dealing with one's family, profession and society.

The best promoter of sleep is a healthy way of life. This can be aided by soporific medicinal herbs of valerian, hops, lemon balm, angelica, St. John's wort, etc.

The presence of older people who supplement the youthful powers of the younger population with the wisdom and knowledge of age is of great significance for the culture of all peoples. For this reason people of this age also require a healthy and healthfully maintained way of life!

II. Recipes

JUICES*

Juices are uncooked food rich in vitamins and minerals in a form which is liquidized by some mechanical means; they are meant to be a special enrichment to the diet. They are of considerable value in cases where roughage (cellulose) must be avoided, or in the case of gastro-intestinal conditions.

It should, however, be realized that the whole fruit and vegetable are, without exception, of greater value, and in the long run cannot be replaced by juices. As soon as permissible, a return should therefore be made to whole fruit and raw vegetables.

Many types of juice extractors are obtainable for squeezing out the fruit and vegetable juices. These include the small hand model, the juice-extracting attachment of an electric mixer, or electric blender. If the hand press is used, the fruit or vegetables must first be cut up. Before squeezing, apples, pears, and all root vegetables should be finely grated; leaf vegetables and herbs should be finely chopped.

Note: If there is no opportunity to prepare juice at home, high-value bottled grape , fruit and vegetable juice can be obtained at the health food store.

1. Fruit Juices

Serve immediately after extracting. Delay of any kind causes loss in value.

a) Unmixed Fruit Juices (without any addition)

Oranges, tangerines, grapefruit, apples, pears, grapes, strawberries, raspberries, red currants, blueberries, peaches, apricots, plums.

b) Mixed Fruit Juices:

Orange , tangerine , grapefruit , or
Berry juice with apple juice
Berry juice with peach , apricot or plum juice
Bananas, mashed and whisked, with orange , berry , peach or apricot juice
Additional ingredients as required or prescribed:
Lemon juice, raw sugar, honey, fruit concentrate yogurt, almond purée, cream of linseed, rice, or barley (for gastrointestinal conditions).

2. Vegetable Juices

Served fresh, they have a high vitamin and mineral content. Each juice has its own special value (see chapter on mineral substances and vitamins in the Bircher-Benner cookbook, *Eating Your Way To Health,* Penguin).

a) Unmixed Vegetable Juices:

Tomatoes, carrots, beetroot, white radishes, cabbage, celeriac, potatoes,* all leaf, root and tuberous vegetables.

b) Mixed Vegetable Juices:

In our experience, the best mixtures are:
Carrots, tomatoes, spinach (in equal proportions)
Tomatoes and carrots

---

* Potato Juice: Use well-cleaned, if necessary peeled, potatoes. Use no unripe, greenish or sprouting ones. Prepare like carrot juice. Does not taste very pleasant, but may be suggested by a doctor.

Tomatoes and spinach

Other mixtures (and vegetable cocktails) can be combined according to individual taste.

For a change, add to the mixture before extracting, some sorrel, tender nettles, chives, parsley, tender young celery or celeriac leaves or root.

Additional supplementary ingredients

Per glass (about 5-7 oz.):

1 tbsp. buttermilk or yogurt, some lemon juice, fruit concentrate; or cream of linseed, rice or barley.

Other leaf vegetables which may be added include: white or green cabbage, Romaine lettuce, endive, lamb's lettuce, dandelion. In spring, dandelion, sorrel and nettle juice are suggested, to cleanse the blood.

3. Cereal Cream as Supplement to Juices

Add 1/3 cream to the other raw juices to neutralize the tart fruit taste.

a) Rice or barley purée: (constipating)

1 heaping tsp. rice or barley flour

7 oz. water

Stir cold and cook for 5 min. stirring constantly, allow to cool.

b) Linseed purée: (mild laxative)

1 tbsp. linseed

7 oz. water

Wash linseed and cook for 10 min.; strain and allow to cool. The daily amount can be prepared once and kept in a thermos flask for mixing all raw juices with it.

4. Wheat Germ

5 tbsp. fresh wheat germ, divided into 4-5 portions/day.

VARIETIES OF MILK

5. Almond Milk

(A vegetable protein-fat-food; mucilaginous; soothing.)

1 tbsp. almond purée
1 tsp. honey
3/4 cup water or 3/4 cup water and 1/4 cup fruit juice which will produce slight thickening

Mix almond purée and honey together with whisk. Add water drop by drop continually whisking or stirring well.

6. Sesame Milk

2 cups water (hot or cold)
1 level tbsp. sesame puree
1 tsp. honey

Mix the purée and honey with a blender while adding water drop by drop.

7. Soya Milk

1 cup crushed soy beans
7 cups water
water to mix
1 tbsp. honey
Wash and dry soy beans. Crush in nut mill or Mouli-grater or electric blender.

Soak soy beans for 2 hrs. Boil for 20 min. in soaking water, stirring constantly.

Rub through a sieve.

Add water until of same consistency as cow's milk.

Add sugar and allow to cool.

8. Yogurt, I

Yogurt is the purest, most efficacious and easily digestible way of supplying dairy milk protein. It stimulates the digestion.

The simplest way to make yogurt at home is with an electric yogurt maker. Follow manufacturer's directions.

9. Yogurt, II

4 cups milk
1 tbsp. yogurt
Bring milk to the boil. Cool to 100°F.
Whisk yogurt together with milk.
Pour into a glass receptacle.
Cover with cheese cloth and a lid.
Cover with blanket or cushion or put in very low oven.
Leave warm for 12-24 hrs.
Store in refrigerator until required.

Commercial yogurt can be used if a good quality can be obtained from a dairy or a health food store.

Buttermilk is fat-free but retains the most valuable minerals, proteins and carbohydrates of whole milk.

10. Junket with Fruits

3 cups milk
1-2 tbsp. honey
Vanilla sugar or lemon peel, grated
1/2 tablet junket
1 tbsp. water
Fresh berries, sugared
1/2 cup cream
Warm milk and sweetener to 98°F.

Pulverize the tablet, dissolve in water and add to the warmed milk, rapidly stirring, and immediately pour into glasses.

When the junket has set, refrigerate it.

Shortly before serving spread the berries over the junket and garnish with whipped cream.

MUESLI

The original recipe for Muesli, worked out by Dr. Bircher-Benner, should be considered a prescription rather than a recipe. If closely followed it will not only provide the best balance of essential nutrients, but experience has also shown that people will not become tired of it, if regularly taken once or twice per day—something which may easily happen if richer and more elaborate versions are offered.

Any apple which is juicy, tart and white-fleshed is recommended. A combination of eating and cooking apples often yields the best results. For example, any of the following, alone or in combination: Cortland, McIntosh, Rhode Island Greening, Northern Spy, Winesap, Jonathan, Gravenstein.

Later on in the season, when home-grown apples tend to become dry and tasteless, their flavor can be improved by the addition, just before serving, of some freshly grated orange or lemon peel, orange juice or rose hip purée.

Note.—Before preparing any of the following Muesli recipes, the rolled oats or oatmeal should be soaked beforehand for 12 hours. It is not necessary to soak the quick-cooking varieties if they have to be used. They are, however, not so valuable since heating processes have been used in their manufacture. The less heat a cereal has undergone, the greater will be its value.

11. Apple Muesli

1 tbsp. rolled oats (soaked for 12 hrs. in 3 tbsp. water)
1 tsp. lemon juice (orange juice, in case of acid stomach)
1 tbsp. sweetened or unsweetened condensed milk
1 tbsp. honey
1 large apple (or 2-3 small ones)
1 tbsp. grated filberts or almonds

Mix lemon juice and condensed milk to a smooth cream.

Add to oats, stirring thoroughly.

Wash apples, wipe with cloth and remove tops, cores and any blemishes.

Using a two-way or Bircher grater, grate apple into mixture, stirring frequently to prevent discoloring.

Sprinkle nuts over the finished dish and serve immediately.

Note: 1-2 tbsp. water or orange juice can be added if required, depending on the variety of apple used and the length of time they have been in storage.

Instead of 1 tbsp. rolled oats, the following can be used: 1 tsp. rolled oats, previously soaked, and 1 tsp. other cereal grains. These should be soaked in water 12 hrs., then rinsed through a sieve and in cold water, and used either whole, coarsely ground, or crushed in electric blender. Alternatively, cereal flakes such as wheat, rice, barley, rye, millet, buckwheat or soya or dried wheat flakes (possibly mixed with yeast flakes for vitamin B) may be used. Most of these are obtainable at health food stores or leading grocers.

12. Apple Muesli with Almond or Sesame Purée

(Muesli without animal protein: for vegetarians and in cases of allergy.)

1 tbsp. rolled oats soaked for 12 hrs. in 3 tbsp. water
1 tbsp. almond or sesame pureé diluted in 3 tbsp. water
1 tsp. lemon juice
1 tbsp. honey
1 large apple

Stir all ingredients except apple constantly until the mixture becomes emulsified. Prepare and add the apple as in Basic Recipe, no. 11.

13. Apple Muesli with Yogurt–Cottage Cheese–Linseed Oil (or Corn Oil)–Apple–Banana–Orange Juice

(Diet when milk is not tolerated, promotes digestion, antacid, not filling, *protects the liver, adverse to tumors.)*

1 tbsp. oat flakes
3 tbsp. orange juice
2 tbsp. yogurt
1 tbsp. cottage cheese
1 tbsp. honey
1 tbsp. linseed oil
5 oz. apple
1 creamed banana

Soak the oats for 12 hrs. in orange juice.
Mix all ingredients except fruit into a smooth sauce.
Prepare the apple as in Basic Recipe, no. 11.
This muesli with its content of unsaturated fatty acids is especially valuable for old people.

14. Apple Muesli With Cream

(Specially enriched dish for those wanting to put on weight. If permitted by physician.)

1 heaped tsp. rolled oats soaked for 12 hrs. in 1-2 tbsp. water
4-6 tsp. lemon or orange juice
1 tbsp. honey
1 large apple

Add cream, lemon juice and honey to the oats and mix thoroughly. Prepare and add apple as in Basic Recipe, no. 11.

15. Muesli with Berries or Stone Fruit

(Especially rich in vitamin C.)

As for Basic Recipe, no. 11, substituting for the apple:
3/4 cup strawberries, or raspberries, red and black currants, blackberries, blueberries (no sour berries)
or 1/2 lb. peaches, apricots, plums or greengages

Berries:

1. Select, wash and hull berries
2. Crush with fork or wooden spoon
   Continue as Basic Recipe, no. 11.

Stone Fruit:

1. Select, wash and stone
2. Chop up or reduce to pulp in electric blender
   Continue as Basic Recipe, no. 11.

16. Muesli With Various Fruits

Strawberries and raspberries
Strawberries and apple
Blackberries and apple
Apple with finely cut orange or tangerine slices
Apple and bananas
(For preparation of the sauce refer to Basic Recipe, no. 11.)

17. Shredded Bananas

2 oz. cracked wheat
Pinch salt
About 1/2 cup water
1 banana

Cook the wheat, water and salt together for about 20 min. on a small flame.

Cut banana into small slices or into cubes and mix into the cooked cereal.

Note: All these recipes can be finely puréed in a mixer according to the condition of the stomach or the intestine. Follow the physician's instructions.

RAW VEGETABLES

The following four principles must be observed in the preparation of raw vegetables:

1. Freshness

The ideal vegetables are sun-ripened, organically grown, compost-fertilized, from one's own garden.

Raw vegetables should, if possible, be prepared just before they are intended to be eaten, so that no wilting and loss of juice takes place. After they have been chopped, grated or shredded they should not be exposed to the air for too long but should be mixed immediately with the dressing to prevent oxidizing.

2. Quality

Leaf and root vegetables should be young, tender and of good color. They should, whenever possible, have been grown on soil fertilized with compost and be free of plant diseases. This is specially important in the case of invalid diet.

3. Thorough Cleaning

The instructions given below on the cleaning of vegetables must be followed exactly, to get rid of any worms and to avoid infection with colibacilli.

Compost-grown vegetables, and those grown without chemical or animal manure, do not contain any worm eggs.

4. Well-balanced Mixtures

Whenever possible, every raw vegetable dish should combine roots-fruit-leaves. Invalid diet, in particular, should always include green leaves. The dressing used for the same raw vegetable salad should also be varied as much as possible.

Bright and harmonious colors make salad dishes more attractive and increase the pleasure of eating.

Herbs, radishes and young carrots, etc., are effective as decorations when, for special occasions, a more festive air is wanted. Not more than three raw vegetables, however, should be served for any single daily salad, more attention being paid to variety during the course of the day. Too much variety can have a bad effect on the digestion.

Cleaning of leaf vegetables: Boston and Romaine lettuce, endive, kale, white cabbage, red cabbage, etc.; separate the leaves, remove brown and imperfect parts and leave to soak for 1 hr. in slightly salted water (1 handful to about 6 qts. water). Rinse several times, if possible washing each leaf separately under the tap. Drain well in wire basket or clean cloth.

Special care must be taken with the preparation and washing of corn salad or lamb's lettuce, spinach, dandelion, lettuce, cress, brussel sprouts, and similar small leafy salads. Remove any little roots and tough parts and rinse thoroughly.

Halve chicory, remove outer leaves and wash well.

Cleaning of root vegetables: Carrots, beetroots, turnips, radishes, kohlrabi, celeriac and salsify: Scrub roots with a brush under running water. Peel and put immediately into cold water to which salt and lemon juice have been added (half a lemon or squeezed out peel to about 6 qts. water), so that vegetables do not lose their fresh color.

Cleaning of vegetable fruits: Tomatoes, cucumbers, zucchini, green and red peppers: Wash and if necessary, peel and cut up into small pieces.

Peel cucumbers starting from the center, working toward the ends. Cut off bitter ends. Tender cucumbers need not be peeled.

Use only very young, tender zucchini for salad; do not peel. Green peppers are less sharp than the red variety. Cut peppers in half and remove the seeds, score thick parts and soak in water if too sharp.

Cut cauliflower into quarters, remove imperfect parts, scrape stalk lightly and put into salt water. Scrape celery and cut away tough parts. Halve leeks, remove bad parts and rinse thoroughly. Halve fennel and wash.

Special methods of cleaning: If there is any doubt as to the growing and hygienic handling of any fruit or vegetables, or their freedom from bacteria, the following methods of cleaning must be observed:

1. In order to destroy any worm eggs and insects, put vegetables into a diluted salt solution (1 handful cooking salt to about 6 qt. water). The salt solution dissolves the protein layer by which the worm eggs are attached and subsequent rinsing of the vegetables remove them.
2. Bacteria, coli bacilli and fungi, which are not harmful to healthy people, particularly in northern countries, can be removed with citric acid or vinegar. The vegetables, particularly leafy ones, should be left in a solution of 2 oz. citric acid to about 2 pt. water for 15 min. Rinse well afterwards under running water. If the citric acid solution is strained and set aside, it can be used three or four times.

3. Put root vegetables and vegetable fruits in a colander or sieve and dip into boiling water for ten seconds. The outer layer is thus freed of any bacteria while the vegetables remain raw inside.
4. Vegetable and fruit juices can be practically freed of bacteria if lemon juice is added (one-fifth of the total quantity of juice).
5. To prevent any danger of amoebic infection in the tropics, dip the prepared vegetables into a chloride of lime solution (1/6 oz. to 2 pt. water), then wash well in boiled water, to remove all traces of it.

Various Methods of Cutting Up the Vegetables

Boston lettuce, Redleaf lettuce, lamb's lettuce, dandelion, cress, cress, watercress	Leave whole, or halve largest leaves.
Romaine lettuce, endive, chicory	Cut into 1/4 in. strips.
Spinach, leeks, peppers, celery, fennel	Shred.
Kale, white and red cabbage, Brussels sprouts	Shred finely.
Carrots, beetroots, turnips, celeriac (white radishes, salsify, kohirabi)	Grate with two-way grater or preferably Bircher grater.
Cucumbers, squash, red radishes, cauliflower, zucchini	Slice very finely or grate with Bircher grater.

SALAD DRESSING

18. French Dressing

1 tbsp. oil
Some grated onion or garlic
1 tsp. fresh or 1/4 tsp. dried green herbs
1 tsp. lemon juice

Mix all ingredients together thoroughly

19. Homemade Mayonnaise Dressing

1 egg yolk
1 cup oil
Lemon juice according to taste

Whisk yolk. Add oil drop by drop, whisking continuously (the oil should not be too cold or too warm). Add lemon juice when mixture becomes too thick. Season with onion, garlic and herbs.

Note: Above quantity is sufficient for 6-8 portions, or even more if more oil is added. For 1 serving, use 1 tbsp. mayonnaise, only.

20. Mayonnaise Dressing with Soy Flour

(For vegetarian diet and when animal protein should be avoided, soy flour replaces egg.)

2 level tbsp. soy flour
6 tbsp. water
3/4 cup oil
3 tbsp. lemon juice

Mix the soy flour and water to a smooth paste. Add oil and lemon juice drop by drop, very slowly, then whisk well.

21. Cottage Cheese Sauce

4 oz. cottage cheese
Buttermilk
1/2 tsp. lemon juice

Mix all ingredients together into a thick sauce. Season with chives or parsley and other herbs according to taste. Salt very lightly. Especially good with artichokes. Color and taste of cottage cheese can be varied with tomato, spinach or carrot juice.

Note: Use various dressings depending upon the physician's instructions.

22. Yogurt Dressing

(For a low fat diet.)

2-3 tbsp. yogurt
Few drops lemon juice
1 tsp. fresh or 1/4 tsp. dried green herbs

Whisk all ingredients thoroughly together.

23. Almond Purée or Sesame Purée Sauce

(For vegetarian diet and when animal protein should be avoided.)

1 tbsp. purée
3 tbsp. water
1 tsp. lemon juice
Some onion (and garlic if liked)
1 tsp. fresh or 1/4 tsp. dried green herbs (if liked)

Add water and mix all ingredients together slowly and thoroughly.

24. Carrot Sauce

1 medium carrot
1/2 cup vegetable stock
Salt, onion, rosemary, if desired

Mix all ingredients in a blender.

25. Vinaigrette Sauce

1 tbsp. corn oil
1 tsp. lemon juice
1 tsp. water or vegetable stock
1 tsp. cooked onion
1-2 gherkins
1 tsp. diced tomato

Mix thoroughly. Season with parsley or chives and celery salt.

Suggested Recipes for Salads and Raw Vegetables

26. Boston Lettuce	Use whole leaves
27. Redleaf Lettuce	Use whole leaves
28. Endive	Cut in 1/2-in. strips
29. Romaine Lettuce	Cut in 1/2-in. strips
30. Lamb's Lettuce	Use whole leaves
31. Cresses	Use whole leaves
32. Spinach	Cut in 1/4-in. strips
33. Cabbage: white cabbage, savoy, Brussels sprouts, sauerkraut, Chinese cabbage	Shred finely
34. Tomatoes	Slice or dice
35. Fennel	Slice finely and chop
36. Peppers	Shred finely
37. White Radishes	Slice or grate
38. Red Radishes	Grate or slice finely
39. Celery	Shred finely
40. Squash or Zucchini	Slice finely or grate roughly
41. Carrots	Grate finely
42. Celeriac	Grate finely
43. Beetroots	Grate finely or roughly
44. Cauliflower	Separate florets, grate stalks
45. Chicory and Belgian Endives	Cut in 1/2-in. strips, shred
46. Jerusalem Artichokes	Grate
47. Kohlrabi	Grate or chop finely
48. Red Cabbage	Shred or grate finely

Are Prepared With:

French dressing		Chives, onion
French dressing		Chives, onion
French dressing	or mayonnaise	Chives, onion, parsley
French dressing	or mayonnaise	Sweet basil, marjoram
French dressing	or mayonnaise	Onion
French dressing	or mayonnaise	Onion
French dressing	or mayonnaise	Peppermint
French dressing	or mayonnaise	Lovage, savory, thyme, caraway seeds
French dressing	or mayonnaise	Basil, thyme, dill
French dressing	or mayonnaise	Onion, chives
French dressing	or mayonnaise	Chives
French dressing	or cream dressing	Chives
French dressing	or cream dressing	Chives
French dressing	or cream dressing	Onion, chives
French dressing	or mayonnaise	Dill, basil, borage
French dressing	or cream dressing	Marjoram, lovage
Cream dressing	or French dressing	Basil, thyme
Cream dressing	or mayonnaise	Lovage, thyme, caraway seeds
Cream dressing	or mayonnaise	Basil, marjoram, walnuts
Cream dressing	or French dressing	Tarragon, marjoram
Cream dressing		Thyme, lemon balm
Cream dressing	or French dressing	Thyme, lovage
Cream dressing	or French dressing	Some grated apple, caraway seeds, lovage

49. Mixed Raw Vegetables

Chicory with diced tomato–French dressing or mayonnaise
Peppers and fennel–French dressing
Fennel, chicory and diced tomato–mayonnaise
Fennel, carrots or other roots–cream dressing
Cauliflower, carrots or other roots–cream dressing
Tomatoes and peppers–French dressing or mayonnaise

50. Stuffed Raw Tomatoes

Cucumber–French dressing or mayonnaise
Celery or celeriac–cream dressing
Cauliflower–cream dressing
White cabbage–mayonnaise

51. Sprouted Cereal Grains

Wheat, rye, oats, barley (whole grains).

1st day: *Evening.* Wash grains in sieve under running water and put in a bowl. Cover with water. Keep at room temperature near stove or radiator.

2nd day: *Morning.* Rinse and spread out to dry on a flat plate. Keep at room temperature near stove or radiator.

3rd day: *Morning.* Rinse and spread out to dry on a plate.
Evening.Place in a bowl and cover with water. Keep at room temperature near stove or radiator.

The grains should have 1/2-3/4 in. long sprouts.

Specially advised for children:

Coarsely ground cereal grains, soaked and mixed in blender with bananas, honey and water.

Mixed Puréed Raw Vegetables

When the physician prescribes puréed food certain raw vegetables can be mixed together with sauce in the mixer. This is the transition from liquefied to a normal raw-vegetable diet.

Sample Mixtures:

1. One 3 oz. tomato
   Handful (1 oz.) of spinach
   1 small (3 oz.) carrot
   1/4 oz. of onion
   Pinch of marjoram

Dressing: 2 tbsp. sunflower oil, 1 tbsp. lemon juice.

2. One 3 oz. tomato
   Handful (1 oz.) of Boston lettuce
   Small (1 oz.) piece of celery root

Cottage cheese dressing: 4 oz. low-fat cottage cheese, 1-2 tbsp. buttermilk, a few drops of lemon juice and some lovage.

3. 1 oz. beets (beetroots)
   2 oz. zucchini
   1 oz. Boston lettuce

Cottage cheese dressing as above.

4. 2 oz. celery root
   2 oz. carrots
   1 oz. spinach

Almond purée dressing: 1 tbsp. almond purée, 1 tbsp. lemon juice, 4 tbsp. water, some rosemary and possibly some finely chopped onion.

Note: For cleaning and cutting of vegetables, see Raw Vegetables, p. 00. A moderate quantity of chives, parsley and onion may be added to every dish of raw vegetables.

Butter-Vegetable Fat-Oils

Older people need to be specially careful in the use of fats. We recommend:

Vegetable margarine and vegetable fat: Emulsions of natural solid fats like coconut oil or palm seed oil combined with the largest possible amount of liquid oil and seed oil, especially sunflower oil.

Fresh butter (should be used very sparingly!).

Cold pressed sunflower oil, linseed oil, poppy seed oil, olive oil: in salad dressing. Treated carefully, they are rich in highly unsaturated fatty acids, very valuable as a cooking fat because of their purity and more easily digestible than heated butter, for braising vegetables. Never overheat these oils!

SOUPS

The recipes are calculated for one person. In our soup and vegetable recipes we use a great deal of vegetable stock. However, since it is not usually possible to prepare such a stock every day, water, flavored with yeast extracts and vegetable bouillon cubes, can be used. For saltless or salt-reduced diets, salt-free extracts are available at health food stores; they are rich in vitamin B, e.g., glutathione and lecithin.

Cream improves and refines every soup and vegetable dish, although milk can be used instead.

Directions for all recipes marked with a large asterisk *

Instead of braising onions, vegetables, etc. in vegetable fat, braise them briefly in 1-2 tbsp. vegetable broth (thus, the taste of the vegetable will be brought out), then finish cooking as indicated in the recipes and put a small piece of vegetable fat in the soup bowl before serving.

* 53. Vegetable Broth

This recipe is for 4 servings. All others are for 1 serving.

Choose vegetables in season, for instance, celery, carrots, some cabbage or kohlrabi, leeks, tomatoes, celeraic and onions. The tougher but still sound parts may also be used, as well as potato peel.

1 tbsp. vegetable margarine
1 onion
2 carrots
1 cup diced celery or celeriac
Cabbage leaves, spinach beet leaves
3-4 qts. cold water
Lovage, basil or other fresh or dried herbs
1/2 bay leaf
Salt

Melt fat. Halve onion, with skin, and brown cut surface in fat. Cut vegetables in small pieces. Add to the onion and steam gently for at least 1/4 hr., covered with a lid. Add cold water, simmer for 2 hrs. Season according to taste.

Can also be prepared entirely without fat; in this case, immediately add water and simmer for 2 hrs.

54. Vegetable Bouillon

1-1/2 cups vegetable stock
Yeast extract to taste
1/2 oz. vegetable cooking fat
Season with parsley or chives

Pour hot vegetable stock over the fat and seasonings.

55. Farina Dumplings

1/2 oz. vegetable fat
1-1/2 tbsp. fine farina
1 tbsp. soy flour
Pinch of salt

Blend fat. Mix in other ingredients and let stand for 1/2 hr. Scoop up dumplings with the tip of a small teaspoon, drop into simmering vegetable stock and simmer for 15 to 20 min. Season with nutmeg and marjoram.

* 56. Tapioca Soup with Vegetables

1/2 oz. tapioca
2 cups vegetable stock
1/2 tbsp. vegetable fat
1 small carrot, diced
1 small piece of celery root, diced
1 small leek, cut in fine strips
Pinch of salt

Add tapioca to simmering broth. Sauté the vegetables in the fat, add to stock and cook for 1/2 hr. Season with yeast extract, parsley, chives.

* 57. Clear Rice Soup

1/2 tbsp. vegetable fat
Some chopped onion
Small carrot, sliced thinly
Some celery root, sliced thinly
Leek, sliced thinly
2 cups vegetable stock
1 tbsp. rice
Pinch of salt

Melt fat, sauté the vegetables. Add rice and stock. Simmer for 1/2 hr.

* 58. Thick Rice Soup

1/2 tbsp. vegetable fat
Celery root, thinly sliced
Small carrot, thinly sliced
Leek, thinly sliced
1 tbsp. rice
1/2 tbsp. flour
2-1/2 cups vegetable stock or water
1/2 tbsp. milk
Chives

Melt fat. Sauté vegetables. Add rice and sauté together. Sprinkle flour over all. Add stock and seasoning, cook for 30 min. Add milk and chives to finished soup. Season with salt-free yeast extract, lovage, parsley, basil, marjoram.

59. Creamed Rice Soup

1 tbsp. rice flour (about 1/2 oz.)
1/2 tbsp. whole-wheat flour
4 tbsp. milk
2-1/2 cups vegetables stock
1/2 tbsp. vegetable fat
1 tbsp. milk

Bring stock to boil. Blend rice, milk and flour. Cook for 1/2 hr. in the broth. Add fat and milk to the finished soup. Season with salt, marjoram, perhaps nutmeg or caraway.

60. Herb Soup

1 tbsp. whole-wheat flour
1/2 cup milk
2 cups vegetable stock
1 tbsp. milk and 1 tbsp. soy flour (mixed together)

Mix wheat flour with milk and stir into simmering vegetable stock. Cook for 1/4 hr. Put the soy flour and milk into the soup tureen and stir in the cooked soup. Season with salt, lovage, marjoram, chives, possibly nutmeg or caraway.

61. Soy Soup

1/2 tbsp. vegetable fat
Some onion
1 tbsp. whole-wheat flour
1/2 tbsp. soy flour
1/2 tomato, peeled and diced
2 cups vegetable stock

Melt fat and sauté onion, adding wheat and soy flour. Add tomato and stock, and heat. Salt if desired. Season with rosemary, chives, parsley.

62. Cream of Oat Soup

1/2 tbsp. flour
2 tbsp. rolled oats
2-1/2 cups vegetable stock
Some celery root
1 tbsp. vegetable fat

Melt fat, brown flour and oats lightly. Add vegetable stock and celery root. Cook for 1 hr. Strain. Season with yeast extract, chives, possibly nutmeg or caraway. Salt if desired.

* 63. Oat Groats Soup

1/2 tbsp. vegetable fat
2 tbsp. oat groats
Some chopped onion
3 cups water or vegetable stock
1/2 cup milk
Some celery root
Yeast extract

Sauté groats and onion in fat. Add next 3 ingredients and cook for 1 hr. Season with yeast extract, chives, salt.

* 64. Green Spelt Soup

1/2 tbsp. vegetable fat
Some onion chopped
1 tbsp. leek, cut fine
Celery root, diced small
1 or 2 tbsp. green spelt (whole or crushed), soaked for 12 hrs. in 1/2 cup water
2 cups vegetable stock

Melt fat and sauté onion. Add leek and celery root and sauté together. Add to the green spelt, add the stock and cook for 1 to 1-1/2 hrs. Season with salt and chopped lovage (or perhaps celery herbs). Strain or run through blender.

65. Farina Soup

1 tbsp. farina
2 cups vegetable stock
1/2 tbsp. soy flour
1 tbsp. milk
Nutmeg
Salt

Stir farina into boiling vegetable stock and cook for 1/4 hr. Add milk, salt and nutmeg to the soup tureen and pour soup over. Season with yeast extract, finely chopped caraway, perhaps some nutmeg, chives or a clove.

* 66. Tomato Soup I

1/2 tbsp. vegetable fat
Some onion
2 tbsp. small carrots
Celery root
Leek
Clove of garlic
Some rosemary
1 tomato
1 tbsp. whole-wheat flour
2-1/2 cups vegetable stock
Tomato purêe (opt.)

Cut onion, carrots, leek and garlic finely and sauté. Add tomato. Sprinkle with flour. Add stock, cook for 1/2 hr. and strain. Season with salt, a clove, chives, bay leaf. A tbsp. of rice or tapioca may be added.

67. Tomato Soup II

4 ripe summer tomatoes
1 tsp. lemon juice or sugar (opt.)
2 tbsp. skimmed milk or buttermilk

Slice the tomatoes, cook quickly and strain. Add lemon juice or milk and serve soup hot or cold.

* 68. Carrot Soup

1/2 tbsp. vegetable fat
Some onion
1 sliced carrot
1-1/2 tbsp. whole-wheat flour
2 cups vegetable stock
1/2 cup milk
1 tsp. caraway
Celery or lovage

Melt fat, sauté onions and carrots. Sprinkle flour over mixture and sauté lightly. Add stock and milk. Cook for 1/2 hr. Strain. Season with rosemary or marjoram, salt.

* 69. Chervil Soup

1/2 tbsp. vegetable fat
Some onion
1 medium potato, diced
1/2 tbsp. whole-wheat flour
2 cups vegetable stock
1 tbsp. chervil, chopped
1 tbsp. milk
Salt

Melt fat. Sauté onion. Add diced potatoes and sauté, sprinkling flour over the mixture. Add stock and cook for 1/2 hr. Strain. Place chervil and milk into tureen and pour soup over. Salt to taste.

70. Spring Soup

1/2 tbsp. vegetable fat
1 tbsp. whole-wheat flour
2 cups water or vegetable stock
Some onion
1 tbsp. young carrot or spinach leaves*
1/2 cup milk

Melt fat, brown flour lightly, add water and cook for 1/2 hr. Chop onion, herbs and vegetables. Add soup and simmer for a few minutes. Add milk and serve. Season with lovage, sorrel, wood nettles or dandelion leaves, salt.

---

* Omit in case of diarrhea.

* 71. Potato Soup with Leek

1/2 tbsp. vegetable fat
1/2 leek, shredded finely
1/2 tbsp. whole-wheat flour
2 cups vegetable stock
1 medium potato, cut into small pieces

Sauté leek well in fat. Sprinkle flour over it. Add stock and potato. Simmer for a few minutes. Season with yeast extract, marjoram, salt.

* 72. Minestrone Soup

1/2 tbsp. vegetable fat
Some onion
2 tbsp. leek, finely sliced
Celery leaves, finely sliced small
1 plateful spinach beet leaves
3 cups water or vegetable stock
1 tbsp. lovage or thyme
1/2 clove of garlic
1/2 oz. whole-wheat, pasta or rice
1/4 oz. butter

Sauté onion and leek. Add vegetable and braise. Add stock and cook for 1/2 hr. Add butter to enrich flavor. Season with parsley, chives, salt.

COOKED VEGETABLES

It is important that very little salt be used at all meals. Herb seasoning can partially or completely replace salt, if necessary.

Vegetables should be served plain. Suitable vegetables are lettuce, chicory, and Belgian endive, fennel, carrots, tomatoes, zucchini, red beets, eggplant, artichokes, because they do not cause flatulence. Cabbages, legumes and spinach should only be used when the digestive organs are in perfect condition.

Vegetables served plain are braised in a little fat-free vegetable broth–cook to reduce the vegetable broth, do not pour it away–then cut vegetables, depending upon the type of vegetable and serve with or without butter or vegetable fat and herbs.

Two vegetables that need a large amount of water for cooking are artichokes and corn:

73. Artichokes

1-2 artichokes
1/2 tsp. lemon juice
2 cups water

Prepare artichokes by cutting off stalks and removing hard outer leaves. Cut off tips of other leaves. Halve, cut out choke, wash well. Rub out surfaces with lemon juice. Bring water to the boil, add artichokes and salt, and cook until tender (3/4 hr. approx.). Drain, arrange on a hot dish covered with a napkin. Serve with Cottage Cheese Dressing or Vinaigrette.

74. Corn on the Cob

(Chew well, otherwise it is difficult to digest.)

1-2 corn cobs
2 cups salted water

Choose only ears with kernels that are tender and milky. Remove leaves and silk. Boil until tender (10-20 min.). Arrange on a hot dish covered with a napkin, serve with vegetable margarine or cottage cheese.

75. Chopped Spinach

(Not to be eaten with tendency to diarrhea.)
Select spinach carefully, throw away the thickest stalks. Wash thoroughly.

1 cup vegetable stock
7 oz. spinach
1/2 tbsp. vegetable fat
Little chopped onion
Some garlic, salt
1 tbsp. flour
1 cup raw spinach

Melt fat, sauté onion and garlic and cook for 1/4 hr. in stock. Add spinach and heat briefly. Thicken the liquid with flour, and heat. Finely mince raw spinach and add before serving. Season with peppermint leaves, sage, fresh butter.

76. Baked Romaine Lettuce

1 Romaine lettuce
4 cups water
1/2 tbsp. vegetable fat
1/2 cup vegetable stock
Salt

Halve and wash the lettuce. Cook gently in salted water. When partly cooked but still firm put into a colander to drain. Place in a baking dish. Melt fat, sauté onion in it until golden and pour over lettuce. Add stock and bake in medium oven 30-40 minutes.

77. Baked Endive

1 large head endive

Prepare as for Romaine lettuce, Recipe, no. 76.

78. Chicory

2 heads chicory, prepared
1/2 tbsp. vegetable fat
2 tbsp. milk
1 tbsp. vegetable stock
Some vegetable fat

Make crosswise incision in chicory stalks. Heat cooking fat in a heavy saucepan and put in chicory in layers. Add milk and stock, cover and cook gently for 1/2 hr. Add vegetable fat to prepared chicory. Season with marjoram and salt. Belgian Endives may also be prepared this way.

79. Stalks of Spinach Beet

3 stalks spinach beet, prepared
1/2 tbsp. vegetable fat
1/2 onion, chopped
1/4 cup vegetable broth
Some lemon juice or cream
Pinch salt

Cut stalks into 2-inch pieces. Sauté briefly in the fat. Add stock, lemon juice and salt and cook over a low flame until tender, 1/2-3/4 hr. Season with tarrajon, clove, parsley and chives.

80. Celery

3-4 stalks of (prepared) celery
1/2 tbsp. vegetable fat
1/2 onion chopped
1/2 cup vegetable stock
2 tbsp. milk or a little lemon juice

Cut celery into 3-inch pieces. Melt fat, sauté celery and onion briefly. Add stock and milk, cook for 1/2-3/4 hr. Season with celery leaves, vegetable fat, salt.

81. Fennel

1 large or 2 small fennel
1/2 tbsp. vegetable fat
Some onion
1/2 cup vegetable stock
2 tbsp. milk or lemon juice
1/2 tbsp. flour

Halve fennel, place in pan. Briefly sauté onion. Add fennel and sauté all together. Add stock, cook until tender. Heat flour and milk or lemon juice and pour over fennel.

82. Swiss Chard

2-3 stalks chard
1/2 tbsp. vegetable fat
Some lemon juice
1/2 cup vegetable broth

Prepare chard, cut stalks into 4-inch pieces, put in the pan. Cover with melted fat. Cook until tender, 3/4-1 hr. Arrange on a plate, sprinkle with crumbs and with fresh, melted butter or vegetable fat. Season with lovage.

83. Steamed Carrots

1/2 tbsp. vegetable fat
1/2 small onion
3-4 carrots in slices or strips
1/2 cup vegetable stock

Brown onion quickly in the fat. Add carrots and stock. Cook for 1/2-3/4 hr. until soft. Season with marjoram or rosemary.

84. Peas and Carrots

(Avoid peas if they cause flatulence!)

1/4 tbsp. vegetable fat
Some onion
4 oz. peas, shelled
1/2 cup vegetable stock
1/4 tbsp. vegetable fat
Some onion
6 oz. carrots, peeled
1/2 cup vegetable stock

Melt fat for the peas, sauté onion in it. Add peas, stock and seasoning, and simmer until cooked. Melt fat for the carrots, sauté onion in it. Add carrots, stock and seasoning and simmer until cooked. Mix peas and carrots in one saucepan or arrange alternately on a serving dish.

85. Peas, French Style

1/2 tbsp. vegetable fat
1/2 onion
1/4 Boston or Romaine lettuce (finely shredded)
5-7 oz. peas, shelled
1/2 cup vegetable fat
1/2 oz. fresh butter mixed with 1 tbsp. flour

Sauté onion and lettuce in fat. Add peas and stock and simmer gently until peas are tender. Add a mixture of butter and flour to thicken liquid. Season with chives, marjoram, salt.

86. Steamed Chinese Peas

1/2 tbsp. vegetable fat
1/2 onion, chopped
7 oz. Chinese peas, prepared
1/2 cup vegetable stock
Some parsley or lovage

Melt fat and sauté onion in it. Add sugarpeas, salt and sauté all together. Add vegetable stock and herbs, cover and simmer 1/2-1 hr. (if preferred the herbs can be sprinkled over the finished dish). Season with chives, marjoram, thyme, salt; add fresh butter.

87. Green Beans

(Avoid in case of flatulence!)

1/2 tbsp. vegetable fat
1/2 onion, chopped
Some garlic
1/2 lb. beans
Savory
Parsley
1/2 cup vegetable stock, or 1-2 tomatoes, diced

Melt fat and sauté onion and garlic in it. Add beans and sauté together. Add stock and herbs, cover and cook gently for 1 hr. In place of vegetable stock diced tomatoes can be used, adding a little stock if too dry.

88. Steamed Celeriac

1/2 tbsp. vegetable fat
1/2 onion
1/2 celeriac, prepared
1/2 cup vegetable stock

Melt fat and sauté onion in it. Cut celeriac into thin small slices. Sauté with the onion. Add vegetable stock and cook until tender (1/2-3/4 hr.). Season with lemon, marjoram, and salt to taste.

89. Celeriac Slices

1 medium celeriac, cut into quarters
1/4 cup milk
2 cups water

Cook celeriac with milk and water until tender. Cut into 1/2-inch slices and arrange fanlike on a hot dish. Top with bread crumbs and melted vegetable fat.

90. Braised Salsify

(Avoid in case of flatulence!)

About 1/2 lb. prepared salsify
1/2 tbsp. vegetable fat
1/2 onion
1/4 cup milk
1/2 cup vegetable stock

Cut salsify into finger-length pieces. Braise quickly in fat. Add milk, onion, and vegetable stock. Cook over a low flame for 1 hr. Season with lemon, basil, celery herbs, vegetable fat, salt.

91. Red Beets

3/4 lb. beets
1/2 tbsp. vegetable fat
1/2 onion
1/2 cup vegetable stock
1/4 bay leaf
1/2 tbsp. flour

Wash beets carefully, cut off root-tips and leaves about 3/4 in. above roots. Cook in salted water until tender (2-3 hrs., or 25 min. in a pressure cooker). Pour cold water over beetroots. Peel and cut into fine slices. Melt fat and sauté onion in it. Add beetroot and all other ingredients except the flour and mix well. Simmer for 1/4 hr. Blend flour with a little cold water and add to the liquid to thicken. Season with lemon, lovage, caraway, lemon balm, nutmeg, a hint of garlic, parsley, and salt.

92. Jerusalem Artichokes

1/2 lb. Jerusalem artichokes
1/2 tbsp. vegetable fat
1/2 onion

Cook like Potatoes in their Jackets (Recipe, no. 111). Then peel and slice. Melt fat and sauté onion in it, add Jerusalem artichokes and sauté together. Season with basil, salt.

93. Steamed Tomatoes

1 tbsp. oil
1/2 tbsp. vegetable fat
1/2 onion
Sugar
4-5 tomatoes
Hint of garlic
1 tbsp. cornstarch (opt.)

Melt fat and sauté onion in it. Cut up tomatoes and add to onion. Sauté gently. Add garlic and salt and cook until tender. Thicken with cornstarch. Sprinkle liberally with chopped parsley or other herbs before serving. Season prepared tomatoes with a little chopped parsley or other herbs such as rosemary, marjoram, basil or chives.

Note: If tomatoes will not peel easily, pour boiling water over them and leave for 2-3 min.

94. Baked Tomatoes

2-3 tomatoes
1/2 oz. butter or vegetable fat
Salt

Halve tomatoes and put in a baking dish. Sprinkle with salt. Put a dab of butter on each tomato and bake in a moderate oven.

If desired a few more tomatoes may be chopped finely (or put through a blender), brought to the boil, and poured over the baked tomatoes. Season with parsley and sautéed onion.

95. Stuffed Tomatoes

2-3 tomatoes
3 tsp. rice (1 tsp. per tomato)
Vegetable fat
Herbs

Cut off tops of tomatoes. Remove and chop up pulp, mix with rice (1 tsp. per tomato), add herbs to taste and stuff the tomatoes. Top with a dab of fat and bread crumbs. Bake in a moderate oven for about 30 min. Season with onion, garlic, rosemary, basil. Add vegetable broth if too dry.

96. Tomatoes with Scrambled Egg

1-2 tomatoes
1 large egg
1 tbsp. cream
Salt

Prepare tomatoes as for Baked Tomatoes (Recipe, no. 94). Scramble egg, cream and salt together, use as topping for the tomatoes. Bake. Season with chives.

97. Zucchini

1/2 tbsp. vegetable fat
Some onion, chopped
1 tbsp. oil
About 12 oz. zucchini
2 oz. tomatoes
Small onion, chopped
Pinch salt

Braise the onion. Dice the zucchini (with large zucchini, remove the seeds). Peel the tomatoes and cut into cubes. Braise the pearl onions and lastly add to the finished zucchini or finish cooking the zucchini together with the tomatoe cubes.

If too much liquid forms, some cornstarch can be stirred in at the end.

98. Eggplant

1 lb. (approx.) eggplant
2 tbsp. vegetable fat
1 small onion, chopped
Salt
Vegetable stock, if necessary

The eggplant should be washed and cut into cubes and can be peeled if desired. Melt fat and sauté onion in it. Add cubed eggplant, and cook until soft, only adding stock if necessary. Garnish with baked or steamed tomatoes.

99. Chopped Cabbage

(Avoid in case of flatulence.)

1/2 lb. cabbage
4 cups water
1/2 tbsp. vegetable fat
1/2 chopped onion
Garlic
1 scant tbsp. flour
1/2 cup vegetable stock or half milk half vegetable stock
Yeast extract
Nutmeg
Salt

Cut cabbage into four. Cook in the salt water until tender. Drain well and chop finely. Melt fat and sauté onion in it. Sprinkle flour over onion and sauté. Add stock and simmer for 1/4 hr. Add cabbage and bring to the boil again. Add yeast extract, nutmeg and salt. Season with caraway, parsley.

100. Red Cabbage

(Avoid in case of flatulence.)

1/2 tbsp. vegetable fat
1/2 onion chopped
3/4th red cabbage, shredded
1/2 tbsp. lemon juice
1/2 apple, thinly sliced
1/2 tbsp. rice
1/2 cup vegetable stock
1/2 cup grape or apple juice
1 apple, peeled, sliced
Butter
Salt

Melt fat and sauté onion in it. Add finely shredded red cabbage, rice, lemon juice and 1/2 apple and sauté all together. Add stock and fruit juice gradually and stir until smooth. Salt moderately. Cover pan and simmer until tender (1–1-1/2 hr.). Peel the apple, remove core and cut into thick segments; brush with butter. Place on a baking sheet in the oven. Garnish red cabbage with the apples and dot with butter before serving.

101. Kohlrabi with Herbs

(Omit when flatulent.)

1 kohlrabi
1/2 tbsp. vegetable fat
1/2 onion, chopped
1/2 cup vegetable stock
1 tbsp. tender kohlrabi leaves, chopped
Salt

Cut kohlrabi into quarters then slice finely. Melt fat and sauté the vegetables in it. Add stock, cover and cook gently for 1/2-1 hr. Add salt to taste. Add kohlrabi leaves before serving. Add Herb Sauce, Recipe, no. 141.

102. Steamed Chestnuts

(Only for those with good digestion!)

1/2 lb. chestnuts
1 onion, chopped
1/2 tbsp. vegetable fat
1/2 cup vegetable stock
Salt
Fresh butter
1 onion, sliced and sauteed

Slit chestnuts. Bake in oven until they spring open, peel. Sauté chopped onion. Add stock, chestnuts and salt. Cook for 1/2 hr. until liquid has evaporated. Garnish with butter and sautéed onions.

103. Mixed Vegetables

1/2 tbsp. vegetable fat
1/2 onion
2 oz. celeriac
2 oz. carrots
1/2 cup vegetable stock
2 oz. peas or green beans
1/2 cup vegetable stock
Salt

Sauté onion. Dice celeriac and carrots and sauté with onion. Add stock and cook until tender. Cook peas or beans in stock. Mix all cooked vegetables together.

COOKED VEGETABLE SALADS

Carrots, celery roots, beets, beans, cauliflower, Chinese artichokes are particularly suitable for these salads.

(Avoid beans and cauliflower in case of flatulence!)

The vegetables should be cooked until tender in vegetable stock or water and then cut into small segments (slices, strips, rosettes). Dress with a salad dressing or mayonnaise. Flavor with chopped herbs.

104. Potato Salad

(Not for strict diet.)

8 oz. potatoes
1/4 cup vegetable stock, hot
1 tbsp. oil
1 tbsp. lemon juice
1/2 tbsp. onion, chopped (if tolerated)
Salt

Boil potatoes and peel while they are still hot. Slice, and cover with hot vegetable stock. Leave to stand for a short time. Beat oil, lemon juice together and mix with potatoes. Add onions and salt to taste. Season with borage, parsley, dill, lemon balm, sour milk.

105. Potato Salad with Cucumbers

(If cucumbers are tolerated.)

1 large potato
1/4 cucumber
1/2 tbsp. oil
1/2 tbsp. lemon juice
Salt

Prepare potatoes as for Potato Salad, Recipe, no. 104. Grate cucumber coarsely. Whisk oil, lemon juice together and mix with potato salad. Season with dill, chives. Rub salad bowl with garlic.

106. Mixed Salad (For Cooked Vegetables)

Choose 3-4 different varieties of vegetable such as carrots, celeriac, Chinese artichokes, zucchini, beetroot, potatoes.

Drain the cooked vegetables and dice or slice them. Mix with French dressing. Season with yeast extract, chives, parsley, dill.

107. Niçoise Salads

Radishes
1 cooked potato
1 small tomato
1 egg, hard boiled
A few slices of cucumber
1 tbsp. oil
1/2 tbsp. lemon juice
A few lettuce leaves
Salt

Slice vegetables and egg. Prepare salad dressing. Mix dressing with vegetables and egg. Add lettuce leaves to the salad shortly before serving. Season with chives or dill, borage.

108. Rice Salad

2 oz. rice
1 cup water
1 tbsp. oil
1/2 tbsp. lemon juice
1/2 tbsp. onion, chopped
1/2 tomato, diced small

Cook rice in the water until soft. Rinse well under water. Leave until cold. Mix oil and lemon juice together thoroughly and add to rice. Mix diced tomatoes and onion and add to the other ingredients. Arrange finished salad on lettuce leaves or serve in shells. Season with chives, parsley and basil.

109. Vegetable Aspic

1 cup vegetable stock
1/2 heaping tsp.
1/10 oz. Agar-Agar*
Lemon juice
Yeast extract
Salt
Tomato slices
Cucumber
Cooked cauliflower florets
Cooked peas
Cooked beans

Dissolve the Agar-Agar in lukewarm stock, heat slowly, making sure it is completely dissolved. Add lemon juice and salt to season. Pour a little aspic into a dish or bowl, previously rinsed out in cold water. Chill. Top with egg and some slices of vegetable, pour in a little more aspic and chill again. Continue in this manner adding vegetables and aspic alternately until the dish is full. When the aspic has set, turn out and use to garnish salad dishes.

CANAPÉS

Open-face sandwiches are easily digestible and generally enjoyed by the elderly either as an hors d'oeuvre or as a light supper in summer. They are excellent also for teas, buffets and cocktail parties. Sandwiches or rolls can also be taken on picnics or for packed lunches. In open-type sandwiches only one slice of bread or crisp bread is spread

---

* Agar-Agar is a vegetable gelatin made from seaweed. It can be used for vegetables, desserts, sauces, puddings, etc., and is obtainable in powdered form at health food stores. It is useful for people with stomach ailments since vegetables and fruit juices retain their full nutritive value and are easily digestible.

with a filling and then garnished. The fillings can be varied almost indefinitely, the fresher and more colorful and attractive the slices look, the more appetizing they will prove. Whole-wheat bread should be at least one day old so that it may be cut into really thin slices.

110. Basic Spreads

Cottage cheese or
Whipped vegetable fat and yeast extract mixed with chives, herbs or caraway or tomato purée (according to taste)

The open sandwiches can be garnished with any of the following:

Raw grated carrot or celery, or celeriac
or tomatoes, cucumber, radishes, cress, onion rings, gherkins
or capers, olives, walnuts, etc.
or chopped egg mixed with mayonnaise
or cress mixed with chopped egg and some mayonnaise or salad dressing
or asparagus tips with mayonnaise, etc.

See also, page 149 for sandwich spreads.

POTATO DISHES

111. Potatoes in Their Jackets

Yellow or red potatoes are especially good done this way.

3-4 small potatoes
Water
Salt

Scrub the potatoes and wash well. Use a steamer or a wire basket within a saucepan. Fill with water to bottom of steamer or basket. Add potatoes, salt, cover and cook 30-40 min. Alternatively, use a pressure cooker.

112. Baked Potatoes

3-4 small potatoes
Salt
1 tbsp. oil
Butter

Scrub the potatoes and wash well. Score skin on upper side three or four times, brush with oil and salt. Bake on a greased baking sheet 30-40 min. in a moderate oven (350°). Put a dab of butter on each potato before serving.

113. Potatoes with Cottage Cheese

3-4 small potatoes
1 tbsp. oil
1-2 tbsp. milk
2 oz. low-fat cottage cheese
Salt
Chives, or caraway, or marjoram

Score once across upper side of potatoes, bake in moderate oven 30-40 min. Mix cheese with milk, add herbs and salt to taste. Put into a pastry bag and pipe over the slit in the baked potatoes. This mixture can also be used for the baked potatoes.

114. Caraway Potatoes

2-3 medium-sized potatoes (long, narrow)
1 tsp. caraway seeds
Salt

Brush the potatoes and wash well. Halve potatoes across narrow side. Mix caraway and salt, dip the cut side of the potatoes into the mixture. Place on a baking sheet with the cut surface down; brush with oil. Bake in a moderate oven for 3/4 hr.

115. Sesame Potatoes

2-3 medium potatoes (long, narrow)
1 tsp. sesame seeds
Salt

Prepare as for Caraway Potatoes (Recipe, no. 114.).

116. Potatoes in Vegetable Stock

Cubed leeks, celery and carrots are cooked with the potatoes.

1/2 lb. potatoes
1/2-1 cups vegetable stock
Salt
1/2 oz. vegetable fat

Wash potatoes, peel and cut into halves or pieces. Cook with vegetables until tender. Add salt if necessary. Add fat to the cooked potatoes. Season with lovage, some thyme, bay leaf.

117. Parsley Potatoes

1/2 lb. potatoes
Salt
1 tbsp. vegetable fat
A little water
1 tbsp. parsley, chopped

Wash and peel potatoes, cut into four lengthwise. Steam potatoes in a wire basket or steamer. Melt fat and mix with parsley, add to potatoes.

118. Potato Snow

4 potatoes
A little water
Salt

Wash and peel potatoes, cut into small pieces. Steam or boil in a little water, with salt, until cooked. Force through a sieve or colander on to a warm dish. Season with thinly sliced tomatoes.

119. Mashed Potatoes

4 potatoes
Water
Salt
1/2 oz. vegetable fat
1/2 cup milk
Nutmeg

Peel potatoes, cut into small pieces. Steam or boil in a little water until tender. Melt fat and heat with the milk in a second saucepan. Force hot, cooked potatoes through a sieve or colander (or mash with a wooden spoon) into this saucepan. Mash all together thoroughly, salt. Arrange on a hot dish; make patterns with a knife, dipped in hot water. Season with finely chopped marjoram, grated caraway and dried tomatoes.

120. Potato Balls

4 potatoes
1/2 cup milk
Salt nutmeg
1/2 oz. vegetable fat

Prepare mashed potatoes. Mix with milk. Dip small ladle into hot water. Scoop out balls of potato and place on a hot dish. Season with vegetable fat, salt, nutmeg.

121. Browned Potatoes

2 small potatoes
Water
Salt
1/2 cup vegetable stock
1/2 tbsp. vegetable fat (melted)
1-2 tbsp. milk
Salt

Peel potatoes, cut in half and parboil in a little water. Put in a deep roasting pan with the cut surfaces down. Pour vegetable stock and the melted fat over potatoes and braise in moderate oven until the vegetable stock has been absorbed. Pour milk over and continue roasting until the cut surfaces brown. Arrange on a hot dish with cut sides up, sprinkle with chopped parsley. Season with nutmeg, thyme.

122. Princess Potatoes

3 potatoes
Water
1 tbsp. cottage cheese
1-1/2 tbsp. vegetable fat
1/2 cup milk
1 tbsp. soy flour
2 tbsp. milk
Butter or vegetable fat
Salt

Cook potatoes, peel and cut into thick slices. Put into a baking dish, sprinkle each layer with cheese. Pour hot vegetable fat and 1/2 cup milk over the potatoes. Bake in hot oven 10 min. Mix soy flour and milk, add salt and pour over potatoes. Put dabs of butter on the top and bake for a further 10-15 min. Season with nutmeg and chopped marjoram.

123. Potato Cakes with Spinach

1 large potato
1/2 cup vegetable stock
Salt
1/2 lb. spinach
Vegetable fat

Peel potato and cut lengthwise into approx. 1/2-in. slices. Cook potato carefully until tender, place on a greased baking sheet. Cook spinach as in Recipe, no. 75, and heap onto potato slices. Put dabs of fat on top. Bake in moderate oven for a few minutes. Season with parsley, chives, nutmeg.

GRAIN DISHES

124. Risotto

3 oz. brown rice*
7 oz. vegetable stock or water
1/2 oz. vegetable fat
Salt

Cook rice in stock for 30-40 min. Mix in fat and salt using a fork. Season with fresh herbs and rosemary.

125. Saffron Rice

Prepare as for Risotto, but add a pinch of saffron powder dissolved in bouillon. Season with fresh herbs and rosemary.

---

* Follow package directions for the exact cooking time, which will vary with the type of rice.

126. Créole Rice with Vegetables

2 tbsp. vegetables, very finely diced (leek, celery, carrots)
3 oz. brown rice
1 cup vegetable stock
1/2 oz. vegetable fat
Salt

Cook vegetables and rice in stock for 30-40 min. Mix fat into cooked ingredients. Season with freshly chopped herbs according to taste.

127. Rice with Tomatoes

3 oz. brown rice
1/2 cup vegetable stock (approx.)
1 large tomato
1/2 oz. vegetable fat
Salt

Cook rice in stock for 30-40 min. Add peeled and diced tomato. Mix fat into cooked ingredients. Season with rosemary, basil, nutmeg.

128. Rice with Zucchini

1/2 lb. zucchini (small)
Vegetable stock or water
3 oz. brown rice
3/4 cup water or vegetable stock
Salt
1/2 fresh vegetable fat

Slice zucchini and steam for 10 min. in stock. Add rice and salt. Add more stock gradually until the mixture resembles a Risotto. Mix in fat with a fork. Season with yeast extract and freshly chopped dill.

129. Rice with Spinach

(When spinach is permitted.)

4 oz. spinach, cut coarsely
3 oz. brown rice
1 cup vegetable stock or water
Salt
1/2 oz. fresh vegetable fat

Heat stock. Combine spinach, rice, add stock, cook together for 30-40 min. Mix in fat with a fork. Salt to taste. Season with nutmeg and mint.

130. Rice Pilaff with Tomatoes

1 tbsp. vegetables, chopped very finely (leek, celery, carrots)
3 oz. brown rice
3/4 cup vegetable stock
2 small tomatoes, sliced
1/2 oz. vegetable fat
Salt

Heat stock, add vegetables and rice. Cook for 30-40 min. Put alternate layers of rice and tomatoes in a well-greased baking dish. Sprinkle pieces of fat over the dish and bake for 10 min. Season with parsley, lovage.

131. Farina Pudding

2 oz. farina
1-1/4 cups milk
7 oz. water
1/2 oz. vegetable fat
Salt

Heat milk and water. Stir farina into the heated mixture. Cook for 15-20 min. Pour melted fat over the prepared dish. Salt to taste. Season with sugar and cinnamon.

132. Farina Gnocchi

2 oz. farina
About 1-1/4 cups skimmed milk
Nutmeg
Salt

Stir farina into the boiling milk. Add salt and nutmeg. Cook 15-20 min. Spread on board to a thickness of about 1/2 in. Cool. Cut into small rounds with pastry cutter. Place any scraps left over from cutting into a greased baking dish, then arrange rounds on top.

TOPPING:

1 tbsp. soy flour
1/2 cup skimmed milk
1 tbsp. chives
1 tbsp. bread crumbs
1/2 oz. vegetable fat
Salt

Add mixture of flour, milk, chives and crumbs. Dot with fat, salt. Bake slowly in oven until firm.

133. Polenta

1/2 tbsp. oil
2 oz. yellow cornmeal
1-1/4 cups water
Nutmeg
Salt
1/2 tbsp. fresh vegetable fat

Coat saucepan with the oil. Bring water to the boil in the same saucepan. Stir cornmeal, salt and nutmeg into the boiling water and cook over a low flame for 5 min., stirring continuously. Then cook slowly for 1-2 hours. Mix in fat with a fork before serving.

134. Millotto

2 oz. millet
3/4 cup vegetable stock, hot
1/2 oz. vegetable fat
Salt

Cook millet in stock for 20 min. Sprinkle fat over cooked dish. Salt to taste.

135. Millotto with Vegetables

1 tbsp. diced vegetables (leek, celery, carrots; or carrots and peas)
1-1/2 oz. millet
3/4 cup vegetable stock
1 tbsp. bread crumbs
1/2 oz. fresh vegetable fat
Salt

Combine vegetables, millet and stock. Cook for 20 min. Sprinkle crumbs and fat over the prepared dish. Season with rosemary and yeast extract.

136. Crushed Cereals

2 tbsp. cracked wheat, oats or rye
2 tbsp. water
Salt

Soak cereals for 12 hrs. Add 2-3 tbsp. water to the soaked cereals, and a little salt. Cook for 20 min. in a saucepan or for 1/2 hr. in a double boiler.

137. Soya Gnocchi

1/2 cup whole wheat flour
1-1/2 oz. soy flour
1/2 cup water
Salt

Prepare and cook as in Recipe, no. 147. Season with chives and parsley or tomatoes. The gnocchi can be cooked in vegetable stock and arranged immediately on a hot dish.

138. Spinach or Tomato Gnocchi

Prepare as in Soya Gnocchi (Recipe, no. 137) adding to the dough 1 handful of chopped raw spinach, or 1 tsp. of tomato purée.

139. Baked Porridge

Oven-baked, cracked whole-wheat or oats are especially tasty. Brown rapidly in a frying pan; add vegetable stock or water and slowly bake in oven until a light crust develops. Serve with dabs of fresh butter, milk or buttermilk, grated cheese; or with fruit concentrates or syrup (in the latter cases use water instead of vegetable stock).

COOKED SAUCES

140. Tomato Sauce

2-3 tomatoes
Herb salt
Rosemary, basil or thyme
Some vegetable fat or 1 tbsp. milk

Cut tomatoes in pieces, cook till tender with salt and herbs. Strain. Add fat or milk.

141. Herb Sauce

1/2 tbsp. vegetable fat
1/2 tbsp. butter
1 tbsp. flour
2 cups milk
1/4 cup vegetable stock or water
Salt

Heat butter or fat. Add flour and sauté lightly. Add liquids slowly, stirring continuously. Cook for 20 min. Season with lovage, chervil, basil, tarragon, etc.

Elderly persons should use sauces sparingly. Simple dishes, cooked plainly, are recommended.

FESTIVE VEGETABLE ROASTS

These are not as healthy foods as fresh fruit, fresh vegetable salad, whole-grain uncooked vegetarian foods, fresh milk, nuts; however, they are far more valuable than meat roasts and–after the stage of therapeutic foods–should become standard fare in the permanent diet of healthy people. But even in a lunch with such roasts, the meal is, of course, begun with raw foods which are the most valuable part of the meal. This can be followed according to preference by vegetable soup, and then a vegetable roast accompanied by a fresh salad and if desired, potatoes cooked with caraway.

142. Karlsbader Oat Patties

(Serves 4)

1/2 lb. whole-grain oat flakes
1 large onion
1 tbsp. vegetable fat
Parsley, celery salt
Marjoram (any amount)
1 tbsp. soy flour
2-3 potatoes cooked the day before
Sunflower or corn oil

Cook oat flakes in vegetable broth or water to a thick paste. Cut the onion into small pieces and sauté. Mix all herbs and soy flour well. Grate the potatoes and mix in. From this mixture form 1/2-inch thick patties, roll in whole-wheat flour and bake in the pan.

Similarly: Make green spelt chops with the same ingredients; instead of oat flakes use cracked green spelt (green spelt is unripe harvested spelt wheat with a piquant, spicy flavor).

143. Celeriac Cutlets

1 celery root
Batter:
4 tbsp. skimmed milk
1-2 tbsp. soy flour
Bread crumbs (wheat germ)
Vegetable fat or oil

Cook the celery root until almost tender; allow to drain well, peel and cut in thick slices. Make a batter of milk, soy flour and wheat germ. Coat slices in the batter and fry in 1-inch deep fat.

144. Bean Chops

Prepare and use ingredients as for Recipe, no. 142, substituting 1/4 cup white beans for the oats. Cook and mash beans and proceed with the recipe.

145. Viennese Soy Burgers

1/4 cup soy beans, soaked overnight in 1 cup stock or water
Some onion, carrot, celery leaves, salt, garlic, dill weed
Batter as in no. 143
Vegetable margarine for frying

Cook soy beans until soft, in soaking water. Purée in blender while still hot. Add finely chopped vegetables and seasonings. Add soy flour, if mixture is too thin. Make patties, dip in batter and fry until brown. Garnish with parsley.

146. Wheat Pilaff

2 oz. wheat groats or Ala
1/2 cup vegetable cubes (leek, carrot, celery root)
Herbs (basil, thyme, lovage)
Some chopped onion
Salt
6 oz. vegetable stock

Combine all ingredients and bake in a slow oven until liquid is absorbed. Top with melted vegetable margarine.

147. Tomato Balls

1/2 cup wheat flour
1 egg
4 oz. Tomato Sauce (no. 140)
Some nutmeg
Salt
8 cups water
Onions cut into strips
1/2 oz. butter or vegetable margarine

Mix first 4 ingredients well and knead, until the dough forms bubbles; add more liquid or flour depending on consistency. Then allow to stand for 1 hr. Boil the water. Force the dough in small portions through a large-holed sieve into the boiling water and let the gnocchi swell until they rise to the surface. Remove with a skimming ladle. Fry in melted fat until lightly browned. Sprinkle with basil, garnish with parsley.

148. Wheat Burgers

2-1/2 oz. wheat kernels
Some vegetable broth
Some chopped onion
1 oz. rice
Herbs (parsley, chives, basil or lovage)
Breading flour
Sunflower oil
Salt

Soak the grain overnight in broth. Cover and cook in the soaking liquid for 1-1/2 hrs. until tender, or 1/2 hr. in a pressure cooker. Then mince in a blender. Sauté rice with the onion in some vegetable broth until it glistens. Mix all ingredients together and form patties, coat with flour and fry in 1/2 inch oil.

149. Vegetable Cutlets

1 oz. water
1/3 oz. butter
Salt
1-2 oz. whole-wheat flour
1/2 egg
1/4 cup vegetables, chopped (leek, carrots, celery root)
3 oz. vegetable broth
Some soy flour
Breading flour
Sunflower oil

Heat water, salt and butter. Pour sifted flour directly into the water and beat vigorously over the flame until the dough comes free from the pan; allow to cool slightly and beat egg into it. Steam vegetables and allow to cool. Mix all ingredients together and form cutlets, coat with flour and fry in 1/2 inch oil.

DESSERTS

Recipes for 4 persons.

For older people large amounts of refined sugar are very unhealthy, since sugar causes fermentation and flatulence and robs the organism of the vitamin-B group which is particularly important at this age. Instead of refined sugar, use pure fruit concentrates, honey, date sugar and fruit sugar available in some Import Delicatessen stores.

150. Junket with Fruit

2 cups skimmed milk
1/2 vanilla bean (cut lengthwise) or grated lemon peel
1/2 junket tablet
1 tbsp. water

Heat milk and vanilla bean to about 98° F. Crush the junket tablet, dissolve in water, add to the hot milk. Stir well. Pour into glasses or bowls immediately. When junket has set, refrigerate. Shortly before serving the junket, add fresh, ripe berries.

151. Frappée

(Serves 1)

5 oz. skimmed milk or yogurt
2 oz. fresh fruits or berries
Honey, or pear concentrate

Mix all ingredients in a blender for 1/2 min. Serve at once. Juices may be used instead of fruit or berries. The juice should be added drop by drop. In this case an egg-beater may be used.

152. Berries and Yogurt

Strawberries, raspberries, blueberries
Fruit concentrate, yogurt

Carefully select and wash berries. Mix with yogurt. Place in cups or bowls and garnish with some choice berries.

153. Fruit with Cottage Cheese

Red currants and gooseberries are generally too sour for the elderly. Choose oranges, melons, strawberries, raspberries, blackberries.

10 oz. berries or fruit
5-7 oz. low-fat cottage cheese
1 tsp. lemon juice
Some honey or fruit concentrate

Mix berries and cheese. Strain. Mix in the lemon juice and serve.

154. Vanilla Cream

2 cups milk
1 vanilla bean (cut in half lengthwise)
2 tbsp. cornstarch
1/4 oz. sugar (fruit sugar if available)

Bring milk with the vanilla to a boil. Mix cornstarch with cold milk, add to the boiling milk, and bring again to a boil. Add sugar. Stir well, cool before serving.

155. Fruit Salad

Pear concentrate or some honey
3/4 cup water
1/4 cup grape juice or apple juice
Approx. 1-1/4 lb. apricots or peaches, melon, apples, pears, red cherries, or any variety of berry

Prepare a selection of fruit according to the season. Dissolve honey in water, then bring to the boil. Add fruit juices. Slice fruit finely and add to the cooled syrup.

156. Stuffed Melon

2 small melons
Fruit Salad, Recipe, no. 155

Halve melons and remove seeds. Fill with the fruit salad.

157. Fruit Jello

1-1/4 cups water or grape juice
Sugar
1 tbsp. agar-agar*
3 cups juice (orange, berries)

Whisk water or grape juice with the sugar and heat slowly with agar-agar until completely dissolved. Mix in fresh fruit juice and pour at once into glasses or small dishes. Refrigerate until set.

158. Apple Sauce

2 lbs. apples
1 cup water
Honey
Cinnamon or lemon peel

Peel apples, remove stalks and cores. Cut into pieces. Add water and bring to a boil. Mix in sugar, cinnamon or grated lemon peel. Cook until tender.

---

* See footnote for Recipe, no. 109.

159. Apple Compote

2 lbs. apples
1–1-1/2 cups water
Honey
Cinnamon

Peel, core and cut apples into slices. Heat the water, add honey and apples and cook until tender. Add cinnamon.

160. Blueberry Sweet

(Good for diarrhea.)

2 lbs. blueberries
Honey
1 cup water
1 tbsp. flour
2 tbsp. water
1 oz. bread cubes
1 oz. vegetable fat

Wash fruit. Cook 5-10 min. in water with sugar. Blend flour with water, add to blueberries and bring to a boil. Put into serving dish. Fry bread cubes in fat and use as a garnish.

161. Strawberry Cup

1 lb. strawberries
4 oz. fruit concentrate
1 tbsp. low-fat cottage cheese
1 tbsp. yogurt

Mix all ingredients together and put through a sieve or blender. Garnish with whole berries.

Note: Other fruit may be prepared in the same manner.

162. Vanilla Fruit Cup

Pears, apricots, cherries and berries

1 lb. fruit
1 cup water
Honey
1/2 serving Vanilla Cream (no. 154)

Prepare a compote of fruit, sugar and water. Pour cream over prepared dish.

163. Stuffed Apple

4 large or 8 small apples

The apples may be baked plain, or with the following

FILLING:

2 tbsp. currants
1 tbsp. cream
Honey
Grated peel of 1 lemon
1/2 oz. vegetable fat
1/2-1 cup apple juice

Wipe fruit, core and make an incision round the apple skin. Mix currants, cream, honey and lemon. Put apples into a baking dish and fill centers with mixture. Put dabs of fat onto the fruit. Pour in apple juice to a depth of about 1/2 in., bake 20-30 min.

164. Strawberry or Raspberry Cream

11 oz. berries
1 cup milk
1 vanilla bean (cut in half lengthwise)
1 tbsp. cornstarch
1/4 oz. sugar

Mix berries and milk. Strain and cook together with the vanilla. Mix flour and cold milk, stir with the sugar into the cooking mixture. Cook together and leave to cool.

165. Apple Cream

1 cup milk
1/2 vanilla bean
1 tbsp. cornstarch
1 tbsp. milk
Sugar
14 oz. apples
1/4 water or apple juice
Grated lemon peel
Sugar

Prepare cream as for Vanilla Cream (Recipe, no. 154). Prepare Apple Compote (no. 159) using the apples, water, peel and sugar. Mix into the cream.

166. Orange Cream (Cold Whipped)

1 piece orange peel
1/2 cup water
2 scant tsp. powdered agar- agar
1 cup orange juice
Honey
1 tsp. lemon juice
1 egg

Whisk peel, water and agar- agar together. Heat gently until the Agar-Agar is completely dissolved. Stir in orange juice and honey. Beat egg with lemon juice together; add to fruit cream. Pour into serving dish. Leave to stand for 1 hr.

167. Lemon Cream (Cold Whipped)

(If lemon is tolerated.)

1 piece lemon peel
3/4 cup water
2 scant tsp. powdered agar- agar
3-4 tbsp. lemon juice
2-3 tbsp. honey

Prepare as for Orange Cream, Recipe, no. 166.

168. Orange Molds

1-1/4 cups orange juice
1/2 tbsp. agar- agar
1/2 tbsp. honey
3/4 extra cup orange juice

Whisk agar-agar into orange juice; add sugar. Heat slowly over gentle heat until agar-agar is completely dissolved (do not allow to boil). Add the other cup of orange juice. Pour into individual molds previously rinsed out in cold water. Leave in a cool place to set.

169. Vanilla Sauce

1-1/4 cups milk
1/2 vanilla bean
1/4 oz. sugar
1 tsp. cornstarch

Prepare as for Vanilla Cream, (Recipe, no. 154).

170. Almond Milk Sauce

1-3/4 cups milk
2 oz. almonds, peeled, grated
1/2 oz. sugar
1 tbsp. cornstarch
2 tbsp. water

Add almonds and sugar to milk and bring to a boil. Mix cornstarch with water, then add to the boiling milk, stirring all the time.

171. Rose Hip Sauce

2-1/2 oz. rose hip purée
3/4 cup water or grape juice
Honey
Lemon juice (opt.)

Bring purée water and honey to a boil. Add lemon if used.

172. Farina Molds

5 oz. farina
6 cups milk
Salt
2-3 tbsp. sugar
1 grated peel of lemon
1 egg
1 oz. raisins

Cook farina as in recipe for Farina Pudding, (Recipe, no. 131). Add sugar last of all. Beat egg. Mix with cooked farina; add peel and raisins. Fill molds, previously rinsed in cold water. Cool, turn out when set. Serve with raspberry syrup.

173. Rice and Lemon Pudding

3-3/4 cups water
Juice of 1 lemon
Chopped lemon peel
Honey
5 oz. rice
Salt

Bring water to the boil with lemon juice, peel, honey and salt. Add rice, cook for 1/2 hr., cool. Fill mold, previously rinsed in cold water. Put in a cool place to set.

174. Red Fruit Shape

3 cups blackberry, raspberry or strawberry juice
1-1/4 cups red grape juice or water
2-1/2 oz. farina
1 tbsp. cornstarch

Boil juices together. Stir in farina and cornstarch. Cook for 10 min. Rinse mold in cold water. Fill and leave in cool place to set. Serve with Vanilla Sauce (Recipe, no. 169).

175. Cottage Cheese Pudding

(When permitted by doctor.)

1-1/2 oz. vegetable fat
4 tbsp. flour
1-1/4 cups milk, hot
1 lb. cottage cheese
1 egg
2-1/2–3 oz. fruit concentrate
1-1/2 oz. raisins
Grated lemon peel

Melt fat, sauté flour in it. Add salt. Add hot milk and cook for a few minutes. Mix in cheese and egg, then add other ingredients. Grease a deep baking dish and pour mixture into it. Bake in moderate oven for 30-40 min.

176. Rolled Oat Biscuits

(For festive occasions, when permitted by doctor.)

7 oz. rolled oats
3-1/2 oz. butter
1 egg
2/3 cup honey concentrate
Vanilla extract
3/4 cup flour

Melt butter and sauté oats in it. Beat egg, vanilla and flour and add to the oats. Knead all together until smooth. Roll out dough 1/8 in. thick. Cut into rounds. Brush with egg yolk. Bake in moderate oven until golden brown.

177. Swabian Biscuits

(For festive occasions, when permitted.)

6 oz. butter
2/3 cup honey
3-1/2 oz. hazelnuts, roasted and grated
2-1/4 cups whole-wheat flour
1 or 2 eggs
Juice and peel of one lemon
Pinch of cinnamon
Pinch of salt
Egg yolk

Beat butter until creamy, add sugar and beat again. Add all other ingredients, except final egg yolk, and knead until smooth. Leave in a cool place for 1 hr. Roll out dough 1/8 in. thick. Cut into shapes and brush with egg yolk. Bake in moderate oven until golden brown.

III. Suggested Menus

Breakfast: Bircher muesli

Whole-wheat bread or crackers with vegetable fat or cottage cheese, perhaps some honey

Fresh milk, herb tea or rose hip tea (unsweetened)

For a change: instead of bread, cracked wheat with yogurt, or sesame milk, or soy milk, or buttermilk or sour milk (when tolerated)

Supper: Bircher muesli

Whole-wheat bread or crackers with vegetable fat or cottage cheese or soya spread

Fruit

Herb tea (unsweetened) or fresh milk

For a change: instead of Bircher muesli, grapefruit

instead of tea, vegetable juice or fruit juice or a vegetable bouillon

instead of bread, jacket potatoes with cottage cheese or open-faced sandwiches with cottage cheese, cress, radishes, tomatoes, etc., or fresh fruit.

Brown rice with green salad

Lunch. Sunday:	Fruit Raw vegetables: carrots, cucumbers, Boston lettuce Celeriac Cutlet (no. 143) Potatoes with tomatoes Fruit salad
Monday:	Fruit Raw vegetables: celeriac, tomatoes, cress Chervil soup Zucchini with egg plant Polenta (made with vegetable stock and vegetable fat)
Tuesday:	Fruit Raw vegetables: kohlrabi, spinach, Boston lettuce Steamed Romaine lettuce Junket with strawberries
Wednesday:	Fruit Raw vegetables: beetroot, zucchini, Boston lettuce Green spelt soup Carrots with herbs Wheat Burgers (no. 148)
Thursday:	Fruit Raw vegetables: cauliflower, radishes, Boston lettuce Artichokes with Vinaigrette Sesame potatoes Orange jello
Friday:	Fruit Raw vegetables: white radish, Romaine lettuce, Boston lettuce Vegetable bouillon Kohlrabi with herbs Potato snow

Saturday: Fruit
Raw vegetables: fennel, carrots, Boston lettuce
Vegetable rice
Apricot compote

Snacks, before and after lunch, are often appropriate for older people who are small eaters and whose body digests at a slow rate, so that they tend to lose weight. Snacks should not be large and heavy, but rather refreshing and stimulating to the appetite, thus, consisting primarily of fruit and foods which stimulate digestive secretion.

10 A.M.: Rye cracker with cottage cheese and yeast flavoring
1 piece of fruit or a little fruit juice
A few pine or other nuts
4-6 oz. of vegetable juice
4-6 oz. of frappe

If prone to constipation: a little dried fruit, yogurt

4 P.M.: Herb tea (peppermint, flatulence tea, Bitter tea)
An open-faced sandwich (see Recipe, no. 110)
1 cup warm milk with honey

Important note: in winter, these teas are warming, relaxing, bile stimulating, and they aid digestion.

DIET GUIDELINES FOR THE ELDERLY

Fat: Refrain from animal fats: fresh butter about 1 oz. per day on bread or served in cooked foods. Vegetable oil according to preference, preferably carefully processed, cold-pressed oil for cooking and for salad. Never heated, cooked or roasted strongly.

Protein: Cottage cheese, soft cheese (low-salt, low-fat), milk, sour milk, whey (best quality protein, valuable for its digestibility, mineral and calcium content). Vegetable protein: Soya, nuts, almond milk, whole grains of all types, potatoes and raw vegetables.

Starch, carbohydrates: Old people usually have diminished digestive juices, have a tendency toward tongue and lip burning and cannot easily tolerate strong spices and acid. They also tend to strongly sweeten all sour things, for taste and to reduce the acidity. Many older people have a "sweet tooth" which severely taxes their digestive organs, robs them of calcium and vitamin B and causes fermentation and flatulence. In order to counteract this, very acid foods, juices and compotes should be neutralized with wheat flour, cornstarch, agar-agar, cream of linseed or rice (with tendency for diarrhea) and a selection of sweet, mild fruits. Use little lemon juice. Bananas and cream can be added to muesli. Honey and fruit concentrate are better than sugar.

Grains: Besides whole-grain bread, grains, groats, flakes and whole-wheat flour can be used in soups. Grain pilaff mixed with fruits or vegetables neutralizes sharp flavors and is particularly well suited for daily high-value food in old age.

Bread spreads: Butter, cottage cheese, mild cheese or oil–tomato spread or soy–almond spread, honey, rose hip puree, etc.

Trace elements, vitamins and minerals should be given special attention because older people – unlike young people – can no longer make up the lack of specific nutrients by eating in quantity. The following is a list of especially important vitamins.

VITAMINS

Type and Name	*Important Sources*	*Properties*
Vitamin A	Milk, butter, oil, cheese, carrots	Fat soluble, destroyed by high heat e.g. by roasting or cooking. Can be stored.

Vitamin B_1, B_2, B_6, B_{12}	Whole grain, yeast, cottage cheese, sour milk, leafy vegetables, legumes	Water soluble, thus often lost in the cooking water; can withstand heat to 250°F., thus destroyed in roasting (settles into the crust of baked bread).
Vitamin C	Fruit, lettuce, rose hips, milk and especially parsley, oranges and lemons	Slightly water soluble. Hashed foods should not be washed further! Sensitive to oxygen, is destroyed upon storage and on cooking in air.
Vitamin D	Milk, butter, yeasts; also produced when skin is exposed to sun	Fat soluble, can withstand heat.
Vitamin E	Plant oils and cereal germ	
Calcium	Milk	
Iron	Honey and leafy vegetables, especially spinach	
Manganese	Leafy vegetables, grains, mineral water	
Phosphorus	whole grains, leafy vegetables, fruit	
All mineral salts	Sea salt	

Less lemon juice when necessary! Garlic and onions are very healthy for older people (in the form of juice).

No haste, no unrest and no anxiety while eating. Dental care, chew and salivate the food well. Many digestive disturbances stem from poor chewing. In case of a great deficiency of gastric acids enzymes may be needed. Consult a physician.

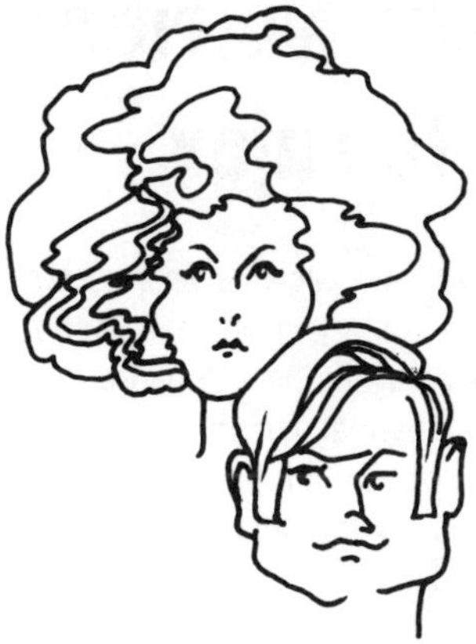

Eighteen Natural-Organic Creme Hair Colors

Natural-Organic Hair Permanents

At long last, Natural-Organic Hair Colors free from analine and metallic dyes; Permanents with no thiaglycolic acid nor its salts. N.G. of Portland, Ore. writes: "Your color treatment is fantastic. This is the first time in years my scalp hasn't been burning, itching, scaling, etc., after coloring—and to think, this condition cleared up with only one application. I am delighted." Write for complete FREE information. No obligation, of course.

CHECK YOUR LOCAL HEALTH STORE
OR ORDER FROM

Randall Back To Nature

7924 IVANHOE AVENUE
LA JOLLA, CALIFORNIA 92037
PHONE: (714) 454-4003

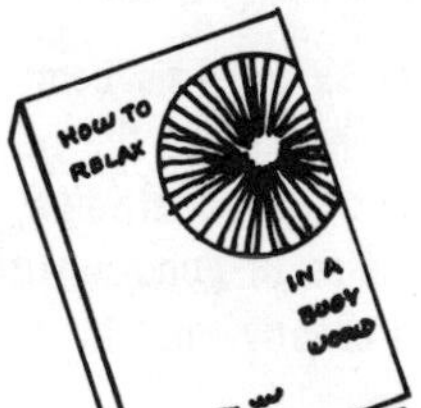

"HOW TO RELAX IN A BUSY WORLD"

Dr. Floyd Corbin, noted blind Philosopher, Humorist, Lecturer, and his many-talented wife, Eve, are both listed in "WHO'S WHO in California." Their message: "Everything can be better for you"—and they show you HOW! New edition, only $3.00.